Although we take it so much for granted, Honey is one of the most important and interesting foods that we know. Not only does it contain most of the vitamins and minerals that are so vital to life, but it has rejuvenating and healing properties that are nothing short of miraculous – 'The Elixir of Life', Barbara Cartland calls it, and in this book she tells of the wonderful effects Honey can have on your way of life, your health and your beauty.

Also by Barbara Cartland

Books of Love, Life and Health
THE YOUTH SECRET
THE MAGIC OF HONEY COOKERY BOOK
THE FASCINATING FORTIES
MEN ARE WONDERFUL
FOOD FOR LOVE
LOVE, LIFE AND SEX

Historical Biography
THE OUTRAGEOUS QUEEN
THE PRIVATE LIFE OF CHARLES II
THE SCANDALOUS LIFE OF KING CAROL
METTERNICH
DIANE DE POITIERS

Romances
THE MAGNIFICENT MARRIAGE
THE KARMA OF LOVE
THE MASK OF LOVE
A SWORD TO THE HEART
BEWITCHED
THE IMPETUOUS DUCHESS
SHADOW OF SIN
THE GLITTERING LIGHTS
THE DEVIL IN LOVE
THE TEARS OF LOVE
A DREAM FROM THE NIGHT
NEVER LAUGH AT LOVE
THE PROUD PRINCESS
THE SECRET OF THE GLEN
THE HEART TRIUMPHANT
HUNGRY FOR LOVE
THE DISGRACEFUL DUKE

and published by Corgi Books

Barbara Cartland

The Magic of Honey

CORGI BOOKS
A DIVISION OF TRANSWORLD PUBLISHERS LTD

THE MAGIC OF HONEY

A CORGI BOOK 0 552 10336 5

Originally published in Great Britain
as a Corgi Mini-Book

PRINTING HISTORY
Mini-Book edition published 1970
Mini-Book edition reprinted 1971
Mini-Book edition reprinted 1972
Corgi new and revised edition published 1976

This book is set in Intertype Baskerville.

Corgi Books are published by
Transworld Publishers Ltd,
Century House, 61–63 Uxbridge Road,
Ealing, London W5 5SA
Made and printed in Great Britain by
Cox & Wyman Ltd., London, Reading and Fakenham

CONTENTS

Chapter		Page
1	Honey in History	9
2	Honey for Love	22
3	Honey for Health	41
4	Honey for Healing	65
5	Honey for Beauty	75
6	Honey for Nerves	90
7	Honey for Happiness	104
8	Honey for Specific Complaints	109
9	'The Wonder Diet'	113
10	The Magic of Honey	125
11	Addresses and Prices of Products	132

Other books by BARBARA CARTLAND:

Romantic Novels, over 150, the most recently published being:

Fragrant Flower
The Elusive Earl
Moon over Eden
The Golden Illusion
No Time for Love
The Husband Hunters
The Slaves of Love
Passions in the Sand
An Angel in Hell
The Wild Cry of Love

The Blue-Eyed Witch
The Incredible Honeymoon
A Dream from the Night
Conquered by Love
Never Laugh at Love
The Secret of the Glen
The Dream and the Glory
The Proud Princess
Hungry for Love
The Heart Triumphant

Autobiographical and Biographical:
The Isthmus Years – 1919–1939
The Years of Opportunity – 1939–1945
I Search for Rainbows – 1945–1966
We Danced All Night – 1919–1929
Ronald Cartland (with a foreword by Sir Winston Churchill)
Polly, My Wonderful Mother

Historical:
Bewitching Women
The Outrageous Queen (The Story of Queen Christina of Sweden)
The Scandalous Life of King Carol
The Private Life of King Charles II
The Private Life of Elizabeth, Empress of Austria
Josephine, Empress of France
Diane de Poitiers
Metternich – the Passionate Diplomat

Sociology:

You in the Home

Etiquette

The Fascinating Forties

Marriage for Moderns

Be Vivid, Be Vital

Love, Life and Sex

Vitamins for Vitality

Husbands and Wives

The Many Facets of Love

Sex and the Teenager

The Book of Charm

Living Together

The Youth Secret

The Magic of Honey

Men are Wonderful

Food for Love

Magic of Honey Cookbook

Barbara Cartland's Health Food Cookery Book

Barbara Cartland's Book of Beauty and Health

Editor of:

The Common Problems by Ronald Cartland (with a preface by the Rt. Hon. The Earl of Selborne, P.C.)

Drama:

Blood Money

French Dressing

Philosophy:

Touch the Stars

Radio Operetta:

The Rose and the Violet (Music by Mark Lubbock), performed in 1942

Radio Plays:

The Caged Bird: An episode in the Life of Elizabeth, Empress of Austria, performed in 1957

Verse:

Lines on Life and Love

CHAPTER ONE

HONEY IN HISTORY

'Is Honey really magic?' Serena asked. She is a very attractive young married friend of mine, who is keenly interested in Health.

'I think it is,' I replied, 'and I believe that everyone who has ever studied the history of Honey is convinced that it has in it a magic ingredient. Although Honey has been analysed for hundreds of years by scientists of every generation, there remains a mysterious 4 per cent they have never been able to break down.'

'How exciting,' Serena exclaimed.

'They know that Honey contains vitamins and minerals,' I went on, 'in fact five very important vitamins which are absolutely necessary to life. These, of course, are found also in other products, but in Honey there is contained, I am convinced, the Elixir of Life. This is the reason why Honey is stimulating to sex, and it is also responsible for its fantastic healing properties.'

'Tell me more about Honey,' Serena begged. 'I really know very little about it.'

'That's the trouble,' I answered. 'We all take Honey for granted, because it is cheap, because we've known of its existence since childhood. So we treat it far too familiarly. It's rather like a friend whom we have got used to, and we say disparagingly – "Oh, it's only you".'

Serena laughed.

'I know that attitude only too well. It means that people don't trouble to put out their best table-mats, they don't worry about the menu, and they always expect you to help with the washing up!'

'That's exactly like Honey,' I said. 'It does so many things for us that we hardly bother to say thank you.'

'One question I am going to ask before we go any further,' Serena said. 'Does Honey make you fat?'

'On the contrary, people in ancient times used it not only as a rejuvenator but as a reducer,' I assured her. 'Honey is highly satisfactory in the reducing diet because it "burns" quickly, while other sugars are metabolized much more slowly, which allows them to be stored in the tissues as unwanted fat. Honey taken sensibly is not only a marvellous ingredient for health, it can actually help to thin you. But naturally primitive people ate Honey and little else. You can't eat four courses, add a spoonful of Honey and expect to slim. I will give you a reducing diet with Honey later on. But first let us talk about Honey through the ages.'

'Yes, do go on,' Serena begged.

'When the ancient Phoenician traders came into Britain in search of tin and lead,' I began, 'They found such enormous quantities of Honey that they called Britain The Isle of Honey.'

'What a romantic name,' Serena remarked. 'I wish we had kept it.'

'The Druids called us The Honey Isle of Beli,' I went on, 'and when the Romans landed in Britain they found that bee-keeping was a national industry. Of course every one ate honey, with the result that the Britons were very strong and beautiful.'

'Beautiful?' Serena queried.

'Yes, beautiful,' I repeated. 'We've only just begun to realize again after all these years that Honey does make people beautiful. You know that I speak on Health two or three times a week to audiences mainly composed of women. After my lecture is over I always walk round the hall and shake hands with everyone present, and it is absolutely extraordinary how I can pick out people who are going to say to me "I always eat Honey".'

'How do you know them?' Serena asked incredulously.

'Because they have such wonderful complexions,' I replied. 'They really have – it isn't my imagination! They have clear pink and white skin, the whites of their eyes are white, their eyes sparkle, and they nearly always have plenty of shining, silken hair. What is more, there is something "extra" about them, a calmness, a serenity, a certain beauty which is difficult to put into words. I think Mohammed knew this when he said, "Honey is the Medicine for the Soul; benefit yourselves by the use of the Koran and Honey." '

'Why doesn't everyone know these things about Honey?' Serena demanded.

'People are either indifferent,' I replied, 'or else they believe the advertisements which tell them that some face-cream or other is going to transform them overnight from having a bad complexion and looking old, into someone young and lovely. You know that is impossible! Beauty comes from within, and Honey is, I am absolutely convinced, one of the greatest beautifiers in the world.'

'You say that the Britons of The Isle of Honey were beautiful,' Serena said. 'I wish we had photographs of them.'

'Unfortunately I am talking of so many centuries ago that we haven't even got paintings,' I replied. 'The Greek historian Plutarch tells us that when the Romans landed in Britain they were astounded by the health and energy of the natives and wrote, "These Britons only begin to grow old at 120 years of age." He did not actually say that it was Honey which was their secret ingredient for beauty, but Pliny and Elder, who died in the famous eruption of Vesuvius in A.D. 79, wrote, "These islanders consume large quantities of Honey-Brew." '

'What was that?' Serena inquired.

'Well, I imagine he was referring to the original wine brewed from Honey, which was called Mead. It was the traditional British drink, and everyone enjoyed it, from the Nobles down to the peasants.'

'I've tasted Mead,' Serena said, 'and I didn't think it was very nice.'

'I rather agree with you,' I replied. 'It has a sharp taste, while I had always imagined it was very sweet. But I think the modern Mead does not compare with the Mead of the old days, which was pale golden in colour and bubbled like champagne.'

'It sounds delicious,' Serena exclaimed.

'I'm sure it was,' I agreed, 'and there were dozens of variations. For instance, Chaucer's Piment was a mixture of Honey, spices, and wine, and Morat was made from Honey, water, and the juice of mulberries. Piment was the most important of the Meads: it was served at banquets and was popular with Kings and Nobles.'

'Was Mead only an English drink?' Serena asked.

'Oh, no,' I replied. 'Mead in some form or another has been brewed by primitive tribes all over the world, in India, in Greece, in Germany, the Slav countries, and Lithuania. They all have their own special name for Mead, but the ingredients of the drink always include Honey.'

'Didn't the Ancient Greeks have a secret wine?' Serena inquired.

'Yes, it was called Hydromel, brewed to a secret formula, and Ancient Greece believed it had great health-giving properties. Pliny records it could disperse anger, sweep away sadness and afflictions of the mind, and transform people of frigid temperament into someone warm and loving. We know now that he was quite right in regard to this last quality; for Honey has always been called "The food of love".'

'Tell me why?' Serena urged.

'The connection with love is, I am sure, one reason for its magic,' I replied. 'Rudolf Steiner discovered that the amazing harmony and happiness found in the bee-hive is derived from the fact that the ordinary sexual life of the bee is suppressed and reproduction limited to the Queens.

"The whole hive is in reality permeated with love," he writes, "the individual bees renounce love in manifold ways

12

and thus develop love throughout the whole hive . . . the bee lives in an atmosphere completely pervaded by love." '

'So you think that food prepared by love affects those who eat it,' Serena said reflectively.

'I've always believed that,' I replied, 'just as milk will not turn to butter for someone who is ill, nor will a soufflé rise and taste right. So Honey has something special to give from the love with which it is made. As Rudolf Steiner goes on to say: "Nothing is better for man than to add the right proportion of Honey to his food." '

'Does Honey help people to make love physically?' Serena asked.

'Of course it does,' I replied, 'but do let me finish the History of Honey before we get sidetracked. The Mulsum of Ancient Rome and the Lipez of Russia were also famous Honey-wines. They were made from fermented grape-juice, Honey and flowers, and all sorts of other ingredients were added, according to what the priests believed was beneficial for their congregation at the time.'

'Really nice medicine in fact!' Serena smiled.

'Honey makes everything taste good,' I answered. 'I have evolved a marvellous drink for people who want to give a party but simply can't afford the terrible expense of cocktails made from spirits. You buy the very cheapest red wine available – I have used a Spanish wine at 30p a bottle – heat in a large saucepan, and add two tablespoons of Honey to each bottle of wine. Throw in two or three cloves and serve as hot as possible. I call it "Mulled Claret", and it tastes like the most expensive Claret one could possibly buy.'

'That's a helpful hint!' Serena exclaimed.

'The great thing is that people really do enjoy it,' I declared.

'You could call it Modern Mulsum,' Serena laughed. 'I expect it does just as much good to those who drink it now as the old sort did. Of course there was no sugar in those days.'

'Weren't they lucky,' I sighed. 'That was why they were all so strong and well. Cane sugar was known in Europe many years before Christ. When Alexander the Great made his voyage of discovery to India, he brought back some sugar-canes which were called Honey-Bearing-Reed.'

'A rather charming name,' Serena commented.

'Unfortunately what it has done to us isn't charming,' I said. 'Even the very rich didn't use sugar until the Middle Ages, and it was not used by ordinary people until the eighteenth century. Even then sugar was very coarse; it was almost black and had a strong treacly smell. But, of course, it wasn't anything like so dangerous as the refined rubbish which we eat today.'

'Which you believe is the cause of all our ills,' Serena teased.

'It certainly is the reason for a great many of them,' I replied. 'In America it is now thought to be the chief cause of coronary thrombosis. But just to finish my history lesson, I was told the other day that the reason Queen Elizabeth I had black teeth, which is reported by all the historians, was that she got a liking for the Honey-Bearing-Reed when it was brought in by her ships. She then used to gorge herself on it, and, unlike the common Honey eaten by her poorer subjects, it caused her teeth to decay.'

'I wonder if that is true,' Serena said.

'I believe it,' I answered. 'When I see small children with badly decayed teeth and I look with horror at the amount of ice lollies, fruit drops, and ice-cream they are allowed to consume, I believe that sugar is one of the things, like nuclear weapons, that should be outlawed by all sensible countries.'

'Tell me more about the magic of Honey,' Serena begged.

'Well, first of all,' I replied, 'collecting the nectar of flowers, the bees transform it into the most ideally digestible source of energy. There is nothing that gives you strength quicker and better than Honey, as athletes have found since the beginning of time. It is known, of course, that the athletes of Ancient Greece all trained on Honey, and when in 1948, after the last war, the Russians came here for the Olympic Games, they brought their food for training with them. It consisted of steaks and lots of Honey.'

'Why don't more people realize this?' Serena inquired.

'The sensible ones do,' I replied. 'When Sir Edmund Hillary got to the top of Mount Everest – you remember we learnt that he had conquered the mountain on the day of the Queen's Coronation – the news was flashed all over the world. His father, who is a bee-keeper in New Zealand, remarked, "It's all been done on Honey." '

'You'd have thought people would have bought thousands of pots after that,' Serena said.

'People hear what they wish to hear,' I replied. 'They paid no attention when the U.S.A. Ministry of Health in 1936 gave the energy value of a gill of Honey as the equivalent of thirty eggs. But I think the first time ordinary people began to realize that Honey gives strength was when divers chosen to survey the wreck of the *Lusitania*, which, as you know, was torpedoed by the Germans in 1915, were given Honey for weeks before the diving operation began.'

'I remember that!' Serena exclaimed. 'Wasn't the ship in very deep water?'

'It was lower than any diver had previously descended,' I replied. 'The pressure of water on a deep sea diver means that he has to be tremendously and exceptionally strong to stand the strain. So, starting with small amounts, the divers gradually increased their daily portion of Honey until they were eating a pound and a half every day.'

'How interesting,' Serena remarked.

'And listen to this,' I said. 'Every time they were hauled up from the wreckage, the divers were given reviving drafts of Honey and lemon. Now when I am talking to people who tell me how tired they get, I always say, "Make yourself a Honey Cocktail." '

'Much better for them than gin,' Serena laughed.

'Gin is a horrible drink,' I said. 'No woman who had any respect for her looks would touch gin. No, the best cocktail in the world is a wine-glass containing a tablespoonful of Honey and the juice of a fresh lemon. Mix them together with a spoon; however thick the Honey may be, it mixes quite easily. Drink it, and instantly – far quicker than any alcohol – it gives one a lift.'

15

'How does it do that?' Serena asked.

'Because Honey dissolves instantaneously in the digestive system,' I answered. 'You have heard the phrase "blood-sugar" level?'

'Yes,' Serena agreed, 'but what does it mean?'

'It refers to,' I explained, 'the sugar content of your blood. If this falls very low, then extreme fatigue sets in and your heart slows down. If, when this happens, you eat a meal, you will feel better, but your body does not quickly get any real energy. You have to wait until the food is digested and converted into dextrose. This produces glycogen, which is what really gives you energy.'

'It's too complicated,' Serena murmured.

'It is,' I agreed, 'but one spoonful of Honey turns into glycogen in a few seconds and it passes straight into your bloodstream.'

'How wonderful! Why?' Serena asked.

'Because Honey has been pre-digested by the bee,' I explained, 'and being naturally fortified with vitamins, minerals, and other medicinal properties it is really the perfect Instant Food.'

'I never thought of it as a food,' Serena said.

'But of course it is,' I replied. 'If you were cast away on a desert island you could live completely on Honey. I dare say you would be rather sick of it after a short while, but you would be alive, extremely well, healthy, slim, and beautiful.'

'I remember my husband saying that when he was in Scandinavia he was told that Honey was excellent for a hang-over,' Serena said.

'Yes, that's true,' I replied. 'Dr. Oluf Martensen-Larsen, who is the leading expert on alcoholism in Denmark, discovered some time ago that Honey is the most effective cure for anyone suffering from that "morning-after feeling". Apparently anyone who has drunk too much will sober up twice as fast and lessen the effects of alcohol in the body by taking Honey.'

'How much?' Serena inquired.

'Dr. Martensen-Larsen,' I replied, 'advises the "patient"

to eat a quarter of a pound of pure Honey, wait half an hour, then eat another quarter of a pound.'

'I should be sick,' Serena exclaimed.

'You could put lemon with it,' I replied, 'but the idea is that Honey, being thick and sticky, prevents the fumes of alcohol rising to the brain, and being a healer it settles the upset stomach.'

'Is Honey really good for digestion?' Serena inquired.

'I think everybody finds that Honey is soothing to their stomach,' I replied. 'Certainly an enormous number of people have told me that Honey alleviates what they call "stomach gas" and reduces heartburn.

'What is more important than anything else for digestion is that one should take Bran.'

'Tell me about it!' Serena begged.

'Four years ago,' I began, 'I had diverticulitis which, I subsequently learnt, is a very prevalent disease in Great Britain, but at the time I had never heard of it.

'I could, however, see on the X-ray machine, which looks like a T.V. cabinet, how twisted and narrow part of my bowel had become and that pieces of it had to be removed. When it happened to King George VI, they called it "short-circuiting".

'Apparently my condition was much worse than they thought and I very nearly died, but my life was saved by the head of the Royal College of Surgeons and, as soon as I was well enough to think, I asked for my vitamins!

' "Let her have them," the doctors said, in the manner of adults humouring a tiresome child.

'But later on, they had to admit they had never known anyone get well so quickly from what had been a very serious operation.

'I came out of hospital after six weeks and was determined to get on my feet again and start a new book.

'I left the hospital with enough medicines to start a chemist shop. They were, all of them, I discovered, made with chemicals and I found on arriving home that the one most warmly recommended contained liquid paraffin, which we in the Health Movement know kills the vitamins in our bowels and is therefore really dangerous!

'I managed to write my book but not one of the doctors who attended to me suggested that what I should have taken to prevent my operation or a recurrence of it was bran.

'After experiencing another blow-up on my bowel which gave me a high temperature, I was treated with antibiotics which made me feel so ghastly that I was determined never to take them again!'

'How awful for you!' Serena exclaimed.

'Someone then,' I continued, 'mentioned casually that I should take bran and from that moment my whole life has been changed!'

I then went on to explain that now Dr. Denis P. Burkitt has come out with the most interesting research on the effect of fibre in our diet. He is convinced that the whole reason for a great many illnesses such as diverticular disease – which I had – appendicitis, ulcerative colitis and cancer of the large bowel can be attributed to the fact that we do not have enough fibre in our diets.

He has studied the whole question and has found that most Western diseases start from the fact that the surplus food takes a very long time to pass through the bowel.

In a test it was found that African villagers who ate about 25 grams of fibre a day took, from the time of eating to evacuation, 35 hours. English volunteers who ate white bread and white flour took 70 hours.

King George III would never see his Statesmen or discuss any Royal business until he had been to the lavatory in the morning. No one today seems to understand that to be constipated is tantamount to poisoning ourselves.

Dr. Burkitt is convinced that the removal of the fibre content of wheat flour by modern roller milling between 1880 to 1900 and the addition of sugar was the worst thing that could have happened to us.

What is more, he proves that two grams – which is only two dessertspoonfuls – of bran per day will give us every chance of a healthy old age.

I discovered this for myself and since then I have helped so many people to feel entirely different simply because they take two dessertspoonfuls of bran with 'live' yoghurt at breakfast.

You can eat it, of course, with cream, fruit juice or just sprinkle it over a cereal, but I personally find it better with yoghurt as, again, I think 'live' yoghurt is good for us internally.

Dr. Burkitt has gone into every detail so that his contentions and findings are almost impossible to query.

'Ulcerative colitis in Britain is reported in about 80 of every 100,000 persons,' he reports, 'while cancer of the colon and rectum has been relentlessly increasing and now is the most common major cancer in the U.S., topping the number of both lung and breast cancer.'

The incidence of bowel cancer in Africa is only about 2 per cent while in England and Wales it is 12.5 per cent and in Connecticut, which has the highest in the world, it is 14.7 per cent!

Since the beginning of the century we in this country, on an average, now eat $1\frac{1}{2}$ large loaves of white bread a week.

'How much fibre is that?' I asked an expert.

'About half a gram a day,' he replied.

Can you see how little that is when we need at least two grams?

It seems extraordinary that appendicitis should be related to the removal of fibre from our diets, but what Dr. Burkitt shows is that slow-moving bowels and the gas associated with a low fibre diet add up to constipation. This brings pressure on to the colon and particularly to the appendix which becomes 'blocked'.

'Inflammation of the appendix,' he says, 'may chiefly be caused by the change in bacteria as the result of an excess intake of sugar.'

So here we are back to another enemy – sugar!

To return to diverticulitis – it is estimated that 30 per cent of Americans have this horrible disease by the age of forty-five and two-thirds of those over eighty!

This is terrifying because it means – as I well know – acute pain in the left lower part of the stomach, nausea, vomiting, chills and a high temperature.

If only I had known about fibre when I was young!

One thing which I think will be of tremendous interest to women who are always worrying about their weight is that Dr. K. W. Heaton, of the University Department of Medicine of the Bristol Royal Infirmary, has pointed out that fibre is a natural obstacle to overnutrition and obesity.

'You are fat,' he says, in effect, 'not, as is generally assumed, because you eat an abnormal *amount* of food, but because you eat an abnormal *type* of food.'

Here we go back to 'You are what you eat'. And how true that is!

'What is more,' Dr. Heaton says, 'fibre requires chewing, which slows down the amount of food you eat. And chewing also limits the food you want by promoting the secretion of saliva and gastric juice which distend the stomach and make you feel you have had enough!'

So many experiments are coming in from all over the world and it does seem that once again we are going back to nature!

Natural food contains an enormous amount of fibre, only it is taken out of it by those who think we *must* have refined white bread and white flour. These two products are, quite literally, destroying us.

'That is really very interesting,' Serena exclaimed.

'I think so,' I answered. 'But one of my difficulties is to try and convince people that anything so ordinary as bran can really make all the difference to their health. People are so stupid they just won't believe simple things!'

'I agree with you,' Serena said, 'but as you say, people are terribly stupid about their own health.'

'I find they seldom reason things out for themselves,' I replied. 'You know no one, not even a doctor, can prescribe for your health as well as you can. You have to be your own guinea-pig, you have to try things out to see if they suit your particular individual needs, and find, by trial and error, exactly what your body requires.'

'I am sure that's right,' Serena agreed. 'After all we are all different.'

'That's the amazingly wonderful thing about the human race,' I said, 'we are different. Of the millions and millions of bodies in the world, there are no two which are wholly identical. This is why a medicine will work miracles on one person and fail utterly on another. It is also why I am convinced that Nature's way is best, and that all these drugs and anti-biotics, tranquillizers and sleeping-pills and what have you, handed out in their billions, are often doing far more harm than good.'

'People become pill conscious,' Serena said.

'Yes, and they think that something made in a factory must do them more good than what is grown by Nature,' I sighed. 'No one yet has managed to produce in a factory the most miraculous machine of all – a living body. Until they do I shall believe that Nature has an antidote for every illness if we can but find it, like the nettle and the dock-leaf. So instead of rushing to a laboratory for a cure, we should first of all try to prevent disease, and then see if Nature hadn't thought out a solution long before it became a problem.'

'I am sure you're right,' Serena agreed.

'Honey is the Elixir of Life,' I said solemnly. 'We are only just beginning to find out what the Ancients knew without newspapers, radio, or television to instruct them, that it is one of the great medicines with which to combat ill health. It is a magic substance which will strengthen our bodies, giving us energy and vitality, and which, moreover, is a natural beautifier.'

I paused, and then I added:

'And Honey is also essential for a man and a woman who wish to make love.'

CHAPTER TWO

HONEY FOR LOVE

'One of the things which worry doctors today,' I said to Serena, 'is that men are beginning to believe themselves impotent when they are still quite young.'

'How young?' Serena inquired.

'A doctor was telling me,' I replied, 'that he is often consulted by men of thirty because they are unable to make love often enough to satisfy their young wives.'

'That is ridiculous!' Serena exclaimed.

'Of course it is,' I answered. 'And the real reason is that men are not eating properly. I cannot say too often that you are what you eat, and yet people go on stuffing themselves with food that really has no nutritive value.'

'I have heard you talk on this subject before,' Serena said with a smile.

'I have to say it again,' I replied. 'We have poisoned the soil with chemicals. The aerosprays, the pesticides, and DDT have, not only in this country but in every country in the world, turned the good earth into a chemical mess which has destroyed Nature's pattern almost completely.'

'How can we be so foolish?' Serena demanded.

'Money, money, money!' I answered. 'Man believes that if he can get quick crops he can make quick profits, and so every year he has to pour more chemicals on the ground and every year we have an increase of sickness and ill health. These, steeped through the streets and rivers and combined with the toxic waste from factories, have poisoned the sea!'

'The Duchess of Leeds, the artist, was very ill the other

day after eating a sole,' Serena said. 'And someone told me that every fish caught round this island has pesticides in it. Is that really true?'

'Unfortunately it is,' I replied. 'I have been saying for years that we have poisoned the sea about seventy miles out, but a little while ago a mercury product from some factory in Scandinavia was dumped in the North Sea and people in Newcastle were desperately ill. The Medical Officer of Health gave warnings that no shellfish of any kind must be eaten from that part of the coast.'

'It is almost absurd,' Serena exclaimed.

'It would be if it were not so tragic,' I replied. 'When you realize that the Baltic Sea is so polluted with DDT that you cannot eat the fish caught there, not even their magnificent salmon, one begins to wonder what chance our grand-children have of survival. And that is only the beginning.'

'We all know about the horrors of factory farming,' Serena said quickly.

'We also know that farmers give tranquillizers to beef-cattle and pigs,' I said. 'They caponize chickens with Stil-boestrol, turning them into eunuchs and making them really dangerous for human consumption. Of course, people go on buying them because they are a cheap meal! On top of which our vegetables and fruit are sprayed with a paraffin–coal-tar derivative, which is suspected of being cancer-inducing, and we put five thousand chemicals into our food, none of which has any nutritive value!'

'What is the result of all this?' Serena asked.

'The result is very obvious,' I replied. 'Add all this to the modern hustle and bustle of business and industry, and you manage to produce a man who is old at thirty.'

'I find that men indeed are often very exhausted in the evenings,' Serena agreed.

'Are you surprised?' I asked. 'A man who has worked all day, often on an inadequate breakfast, a sandwich lunch, and something out of a tin for dinner, is suffering quite simply from malnutrition. He may have eaten a lot of bulk, but he has literally been starved. In fact, if a farmer fed his animals, especially his bulls, his boars, and his stallions, as badly as the average woman feeds her husband, he would not only go bankrupt, he would be prosecuted by the R.S.P.C.A.'

'Don't you think women try to feed their families better than they used to?' Serena asked.

'I would love to say yes to that question,' I replied, 'but the other day I went to a farm near my home, and I was talking to the Manager's wife. She told me that one of the perks of the farm-hands was that they could have as many potatoes as they wished – they only had to pick them up off the ground and take them home. But every one of them, without exception, ate packaged potatoes, because their wives didn't like peeling vegetables.'

'That's absurd,' Serena said crossly, 'but I know a lot of younger women who do try.'

'I think they are beginning to appreciate more exotic dishes,' I agreed. 'Television is responsible for this, but they still make little effort to get up in the morning. A cereal put on the table with a jug of milk the night before is all that, in innumerable homes, the mother provides as breakfast both for the father and for the children going to school.'

'Are cereal breakfasts no good?' Serena asked.

'When you have fasted for twelve hours your blood-sugar in the morning is low,' I replied. 'This, incidentally, has no relation to artificial sugar, but refers really to the metabolism of the body. What one needs when one wakes is to be re-fuelled, and the proper and correct fuel for the body machine is protein.'

'Meat, fish, eggs, cheese,' Serena intoned, like a child saying a lesson.

'Exactly,' I said, 'and in England we have the best break-fast of all – eggs and bacon. Those two foods really do contain all that is necessary to start the day in the right way, with two additions.'

'I can guess that,' Serena cried. 'Honey and bran.'

'Yes, of course,' I smiled. 'If a man, and a woman for that matter, will have two eggs for breakfast, bacon, a cup of tea, a large spoonful of Honey, and Bran they need nothing else.'

'Do you really mean nothing else?' Serena inquired.

'Exactly what I said,' I replied. 'No bread, no gooey marmalade, which often has never seen an orange. No cereals, some of which are chemicalized substances, flavoured with commercial sugar which makes them taste sweet, but which is really detrimental to the body rather than providing it with any form of vitality.'

Serena sighed.

'I am beginning to think you're right, and perhaps people are under-fed.'

'Sadly they are,' I answered. 'And I am convinced that if employers in every factory or office insisted on their employees having a proper breakfast as soon as they arrived for work, production would go up by 10 per cent.'

'Can you see them agreeing?' Serena asked derisively.

'And how many people who work eat a sensible lunch?' I went on. 'They have something out of a paper bag or they snatch a white bread sandwich from a café. Many firms do provide excellent canteens, but they tell me the young are usually reluctant to eat meat or anything solid, preferring ersatz cream cakes, potato crisps, and, of course, the inevitable soft drinks.'

'Don't go on,' Serena begged. 'You're making me depressed. What do you suggest that a man who wants to be strong, and, of course, virile, should have for lunch?'

'Meat! Meat! Meat!' I said. 'The thirty billion cells of our body are made of protein. No one would be so idiotic as to try to mend a motor tyre with a mixture of paste and water, but that's exactly what we do when we eat cereals and white bread, pastry, and all sorts of starch. The cells in our body require protein for repair, maintenance, and long-distance running, and the easiest protein to take, and the most effective, is undoubtedly meat.'

'What about vegetarians?' Serena interrupted.

'Vegetarians will tell you that they manage very well without meat,' I replied. 'But I can assure you that I get hundreds – and I'm not exaggerating – of letters a year from vegetarians of both sexes saying how tired and anaemic they are at fifty, how nervy and how incapable of making love.

'If you wish to be a vegetarian you have to study the subject very carefully. You have to eat protein in the shape of soya flour, and combat anaemia with Vitamin B12. It is difficult and expensive to get all the right ingredients, and so for the average man and woman the eating of meat, as often as possible, is the easiest way to stay young and to be virile.'

'You certainly sound very convincing,' Serena said.

'And here we get back,' I went on, 'to our Russian Olympic competitors, and, in fact, all the other athletes in Modern times who find in meat and Honey the best possible food for training.'

'We mustn't forget the Honey,' Serena said.

'No, indeed,' I replied, 'And we were talking about Honey as conducive to love. First of all, to make love properly, one has got to be fit. I've always believed that, if a man and woman are naturally healthy, they will be naturally passionate. That is why when people ask my advice I give them the right vitamins, but at the same time always, and most important of all, the right diet.'

'And your diet includes Honey,' Serena said with a smile.

'Lots of Honey,' I answered. 'I often tell the story of how I went to a Women's Institute and talked to its members. I told them how important Honey was in married life and how it would make a man loving at almost any age. A few days later I got a letter from one of the women who had been present. She was not very young, and she wrote to me:

' "Dear Miss Cartland, I took your advice and gave my husband Honey. It *works*." '

Serena laughed.

'Short and to the point.'

'She got exactly what she wanted,' I replied, 'a loving, understanding, considerate husband. You see so many people today think that sex is something quite apart from the companionship of marriage. It isn't. Sex is all important in marriage and is tremendously important for keeping young. A woman wants to be loved and made a fuss of until

26

she dies, and she can keep her husband loving her, she can keep him sexually active, if she takes the trouble.'

'Is that really true?' Serena interrupted.

'I promise you I'm not telling you anything which is not an actual fact,' I replied. 'I've known couples who have made love regularly into their late eighties, and I know too that a great many so-called middle-aged, or even elderly couples, get a great deal of satisfaction and happiness out of love-making several times a week. But it isn't always the actual act which is important, it's the feeling inside the people themselves that passion is still possible for them, that the warmth and affection which goes with the urge to make love is not dead, but very much alive.'

'And Honey can do this?' Serena asked almost incredulously.

'Honey is one of the most important factors for keeping people sexually competent,' I replied. 'To begin with, Honey has a soothing effect upon nerves, and this in itself is very important in keeping people young. There is nothing more ageing than worry, nothing which destroys youth quicker than what is called nerves.'

'People today are always talking about "me nerves",' Serena said.

'It is definitely a modern disease,' I replied. 'Fatigue is another thing which is a destroyer both of our looks and our happiness. If we're tired we are nearly always disagreeable. You would have to be a saint to be utterly exhausted and not take it out on someone.'

I paused.

'I want to talk to you later about Hormone Replacement Treatment but let us now keep to Honey.

'Honey, as we've just shown, can sweep away fatigue very easily and very quickly and we have only to go back into the past to find out how important Honey was to the Ancients who were really concerned with sexual virility.'

'Tell me what they suggested,' Serena begged.

'Pliny advised the Romans to eat river snails,' I replied, 'the eggs of sparrows, the tongue of the goose, leeks, and the yolks of five pigeons eggs in Honey with a bit of hog's lard.'

'That's a mixed grill!' Serena laughed.

'There was lots more,' I told her. 'Ageing Romans tried to rejuvenate on frogs, hedgehogs, the penis of the wolf, and the flesh of the skink – a long thin lizard which was considered aphrodisiac.'

'It sounds disgusting,' Serena shuddered.

'The Ancient Indian heroes, noted as tireless lovers, consumed huge quantities of meat, with onions, garlic, beans, and Honey.'

'So here we are back where we started,' Serena laughed.

'Ancient people knew the value of Honey in many ways,' I said, 'Honey-comb was one of the first contraceptives used by women.'

'I've read many old recipes which were thought to be aphrodisiac,' Serena said.

'The most extraordinary was, I think, compiled by Bartolomeo Scappi, cook to Pope Saint-Pius V,' I told her. 'It was called Pie of Bull's Testicles. He boiled four bulls' testicles in water and salt, cut them into slices and sprinkled them with pepper, salt, cinnamon, and nutmeg. In the pie there was also lamb's kidneys, ham, marjoram, thyme, and cloves.'

'Good gracious!' Serena exclaimed.

'Excellent protein,' I said, 'and doubtless His Holiness ate or drank a lot of Honey because it was acknowledged by everyone to be a powerful aphrodisiac.'

'It's funny that few people think about that today,' Serena smiled.

'All the European recipes for potency incorporate meat in some form or another,' I went on. 'Hares and venison particularly were supposed to be sexual fare. I think actually it was because they were mostly to be found on noblemen's estates, and, as noblemen were better fed than the peasants, it was presumed that their virility was derived from their food, which of course was true. But Honey was always added to sex stimulants in Europe, in the East, in India, and in the Arab world.'

'What did they suggest?' Serena asked.

'In the Perfumed Garden,' I answered, 'a sixteenth-century manual of Arabian erotology translated by Sir Richard Burton, it says:

> If a man will passionately give himself up to the enjoyment of coition without indulging too great fatigue, he must live upon strengthening foods – exciting comfits (these were mostly prepared with Honey), aromatic plants, meat, Honey, eggs and similar viands.

'The Arabs were great admirers of strong sexual lovers,' Serena remarked.

'I always think of Richard Burton translating the following poem with gusto,' I said. 'It was part of the life he knew and loved – the smell, clamour, and intrigue of the bazaar, the sharp dry wind blowing in from the desert, the story-teller warming to the erotic parts of the tale, the glint in the eyes of the dark faces of the listeners:

' *"The Negro Mimun, for full fifty days,*
Served numberless girls and gained honour and praise;
And when he was asked to keep it up longer
He did another ten days and finished up stronger!
Now during this test, it was Honey and bread
Enabled his zabzab to hold up its head." '

'Tell me exactly how much Honey a man should take today,' Serena said.

'Well, I think every man who wants to keep well and healthy, and be a good lover,' I said, 'should take Honey in the morning and Honey at night. Incidentally I cured my husband of bronchitis by giving him comb-honey for breakfast and comb-honey when he went to bed.

'He only had one lung, having been shot through the chest by a dum-dum bullet during the First World War. He very nearly died, was in hospital for years and suffered from bronchitis every winter until I married him. After that he very seldom had it, but he never forgot to take his Honey.'

'And what else?' Serena asked.

'Well, I've made a very exhaustive study of what is too often called impotence in men and frigidity in women, and I've found that in the majority of cases it arises from nothing more or less than bad feeding.

'Now we know that it is impossible for people today to have the right food however carefully they buy, or even if, like me, they grow their own vegetables, and therefore one has to supplement their ordinary diet with vitamins and with other forms of food supplements.'

'Give me a list,' Serena begged.

'I'm going to,' I replied. 'But first of all I'm going to tell you about some very new products which I think are fantastic, and which are the first stimulants we have yet found which are not only harmless but very positively beneficial.

'What are they?' Serena asked.

'They are Celaton CH_3 Tri-Plus, which I call the "Brain Pill",' I replied. 'Keitafo Banlon Pills – a Chinese formula for health invigoration and genital function.

'These with the fantastic Ginseng, stimulate and improve sexual prowess.'

'Tell me about the "Brain Pill",' Serena begged.

'You have heard of Professor Paul Niehans,' I began, 'who died a year or so ago. He was the exponent of cell-therapy in Europe.'

'Didn't he cure Pope Pius XII by giving him fresh cell therapy?' Serena asked, 'and rejuvenate a lot of other celebrities?'

'That is right,' I answered. 'It caused a sensation at the time, but afterwards it was discovered that all such cell transplants are most effective after the transplanted organ has been frozen. The cornea of an eye for instance is more effective frozen and kept in the dark than when taken direct from a living eye.'

'And Brain?' Serena questioned.

'Brain powder comes from Denmark,' I replied. 'For over

two years a certain doctor in Great Britain has been treating a mongol child with it. I have seen his medical reports.'

'What do they say?' Serena inquired.

'The parents can hardly believe it, but the little girl is making sentences.'

'How fantastic!' Serena exclaimed.

'It is amazing,' I agreed. 'I myself have taken the "Brain Pill" in a special foundation for three years. Last year I wrote eighteen books and a cookery book.'

'Eighteen!' Serena ejaculated.

'I have never felt so well, so bright, so gay, so happy, and I can't stop working.'

'You look marvellous,' Serena smiled.

'So people are kind enough to say,' I replied. 'My son, who is thirty-eight, takes two tablets a day and says he has never felt better in his life. He too is working harder and for much longer hours than ever before.'

'Poor man!'

'Nonsense!' I retorted. 'Men like work, and the Brain Tablets saved my mother's life. She was very ill and we really thought she was dying. She was ninety-five. But no, she recovered and is now lecturing, opening bazaars, arranging "Bring and Buys", and being so busy she might be twenty-five years younger.

'"Celaton CH_3 Tri-Plus," I went on, 'contains H_3, the marvellous rejuvenating substance discovered in Rumania by the famous Professor Ana Aslan. Then there is a product to help the heart, the Brain powder, and the Intrinsic Factor.'

'What is that?' Serena inquired.

'It is a form of B_{12}. It is something we all make in our stomachs when we are healthy, but which is seriously deficient in old and ill people. Then, however much food they eat and however many vitamins they take, they don't absorb them. Incidentally, we can buy Intrinsic Factor separately.'

'Now tell me about Keitafo Banlon Tablets,' Serena said.

'This is a tonic which is made in China, and the Chinese

are extremely clever doctors. Keitafo Banlon is made on prescription communicated secretly from the Chinese Imperial Palace many years ago which has been improved on and added to by Dr. Banlon.

'When I was in Hong Kong I spoke to Mrs. Banlon as her husband is Chinese and doesn't speak English. She assured me that every ingredient of the pill was absolutely pure and the vitamins were not synthetic.

'It certainly has been proved both abroad and here by many experts that it is ideal for rejuvenation, invigoration, seminal potency and the preservation of a youthful appearance.

'I find that even two Banlon pills have a sexual reaction. One begins to thrill easily, and every man to whom I have given them has been full of praise at their effect on him when he wishes to make love.

'But again I do not think a sex pill is effective unless one is taking the whole team of vitamins which are important to good health.

'You need also multi-vitamin tablets, containing vitamin A, which is essential for male sexual problems and vitamin E.

'Where a man and a woman are seriously worried about their sexual prowess I would advise two multi-vitamin tablets GEV-E-TABS, combined with two to four Celaton CH_3 Tri-Plus, four Keitafo Banlon pills, two Gingseng Tablets, and three Vitamin A Compleat.

'I know that these have a marvellous effect upon virility.'

'Tell me all about Ginseng,' Serena said.

'Ginseng, is one of the oldest medicines in the whole world.' I replied. 'It too is Chinese, and when I was last in the East I was told that even the poorest Chinese save up their money so they can buy Ginseng because they believe it has such a wonderful effect on their health.

'It is in fact very expensive in the East, but one can buy tablets of Ginseng in England which are comparatively cheap in price.

'Ginseng is specially prepared and extracted from the root

of the Araliaceas plant. Korean Ginseng has been reverently used in the Orient for several thousands of years and is reputed by the Chinese to be of great value in preserving strength, vigour and vitality.

'Originally all the Ginseng was kept for the Emperors of China, and we can be grateful to democracy which now enables ordinary people to use it.

'In the East Ginseng is called the rejuvenation herb and it is considered a panacea of all diseases. The sick take it to recover their health and the healthy use it to build up their resistance to diseases and to make themselves stronger.

'When I talked to a very important Chinese businessman in Hong Kong he said to me:

"All Chinese worry about their virility, and Chinese men put their faith in Ginseng. I personally take it every day in a little brandy."*

'What I think is most convincing is that Dr. Kissenger takes Ginseng and the astronauts going to the moon were all made to take it.'

'Supposing a person who needed to feel young again just took any of the products you have just described; would one of them be enough?' Serena asked

'In everything I recommend,' I replied, 'I always stress the importance of taking vitamins at the same time.'

'Which vitamins?'

'That is something I can answer quite easily. The lot!'

'But how?' Serena questioned.

'Vitamins work as a team,' I said. 'I repeat this everywhere I go because people are inclined to take a vitamin for the eyes or a vitamin for the legs, and then are disappointed at the result. Just as you need eleven good players in a football team, so you need all the vitamins to resuscitate and reconstitute your health.'

'But that means dozens of tablets,' Serena gasped.

'No,' I replied, 'it means you take multi-vitamin capsules.'

'Which one do you take?'

* Ginseng *Elixir* which contains wine is now available I find it sensational.

'Gev-E-Tabs,' I replied, 'I find them simply fantastic. If you are young, 2 Gev-E-Tabs a day are all you should require to supply you with all the vitamins and minerals – 25 of them – which a normal person should need during the day. And even if you are taking one of the fabulous special products I am telling you about, take Gev-E-Tabs too, as a safeguard that you are getting every vitamin and mineral your body needs for nourishment and good health.'

'I see your point,' Serena said slowly.

'With men who make a fuss about taking tablets in any form,' I went on, 'Gev-E-Tabs are really an answer to prayer. My husband always used to say "I'll take one capsule a day!". Well, I persuaded him to take two, and 2 Gev-E-Tabs* supplied him not only with all the different Vitamin B's which are essential to every man who works hard, but also gave him Vitamin E, Wheat Germ Oil, Vitamin A (which every man requires) and every essential mineral.'

'I see they are rather large!' Serena said, looking at the Gev-E-Tabs box. 'Are they difficult to swallow?'

'No, they are very easy,' I replied. 'They are soft and slip down with a cup of tea or a glass of water. What is more, they are homogenized!'

'What does that mean?' Serena asked.

'It means that people with very sensitive digestions can assimilate them,' I replied, 'and quite honestly I find them simply wonderful. What is more, all my family take them.'

'It sounds very exciting!' Serena exclaimed. 'Now give me your advice on what two people, anxious to make love, should take every day.'

'I will give you a number of suggestions,' I replied. 'Remember, as I've always said, everyone is different, but here is my first formula for so-called male impotence and female frigidity:

'After breakfasting on eggs and bacon and Honey, take:

1 Gev-E-Tab (new strength).
1000 mg of Vitamin E – the Life, Love, and Sex Vitamin.

* These are now made in extra strength so one is sufficient.

3 Vitamin A Compleat Healthcrafts – which is essential for male potency and affects the semen.

3 Celaton CH3 – the virility tablet.

Ginseng tablets. 400 to 1000 mg.

'Then a meat lunch and a meat dinner, and last thing at night 2 Keitafo Banlon tablets.'

'Surely that would put on weight?' Serena asked.

'Meat is slimming,' I answered. 'Have you ever seen a fat tiger? I prohibit starch, white sugar, white flour, and whisky and beer!'

'Why whisky?' Serena cried.

'It is very definitely anti-sex,' I answered. 'Give the ordinary middle-aged man two or three whiskies and he becomes dull, morose, and sleepy, and certainly not particularly interested in a woman or sex.'

'What should he drink, then?' Serena asked.

'Not too much of anything,' I replied. 'Champagne is a success with some people, but I often think its reputation for gaiety is more a psychological supposition than fact. A little brandy is the best drink if one wants stimulating, and white wines have always been traditional for sex like oysters and celery.'

'Is this fact or fancy?' Serena demanded.

'Mostly fancy,' I admitted, 'but as successful love-making is dependent on imagination, everything which creates an atmosphere of romance, beauty, gaiety, and of course desire is very important. That is why women are such fools: they grease their faces, pin up their hair, get into bed talking about the price of potatoes, and expect a man to fall on them ecstatically. Love is an Art!'

'And the more you know, the more there is to know,' Serena smiled.

'Of course,' I agreed, 'yet any little half-wit in a mini-skirt thinks she knows all about sex and has nothing to learn.'

'And her mother thought the same,' Serena said, 'and that's why there are so many middle-aged men watching strip-tease in the afternoon or chasing blondes in search of their lost youth!'

'How can one really attempt to help people to understand love?' I asked helplessly. 'It is something one has to feel and which is too ethereal and too exquisite to be put into words.'

'I think I would just say be grateful for it,' Serena said softly.

'Older people are grateful,' I replied, 'which is why love-making in middle-age is often more successful than when one is young. The young take physical love for granted and those who are older and wiser know it is the most marvellous experience in the world.'

'That is why once we've found it we must never lose it,' Serena said.

'Therefore nothing is too much trouble,' I said. 'In fact, any sacrifice is worth while if we can keep alive and vital that amazing fusion of two people so that they become one.'

'So we must try to make people understand love,' Serena declared. 'But they do need practical help. I suppose there are other products than the ones you have mentioned?'

'Many experts who have studied sex problems find Pollen most effective,' I replied. 'Pollen is the male sex cell in plants and is fed to the young bees for the first six weeks of their lives.'

'But it's not actually Honey?' Serena asked.

'No, but of course it should also be taken together with Honey. I include it in this chapter because of its success with tired, depressed, middle-aged men.'

'I have heard that in Sweden they are experimenting with it,' Serena said.

'The Swedes were the pioneers,' I agreed. 'They have carried out extensive clinical trials and have announced excellent results from using pollen to treat prostatitis as well as sexual difficulties. In fact, recently Dr. Erik Ask-Lipmark of Uppsala University was quoted as saying: "We are not sure yet how it works, but we know that it does work!" '

'That sounds hopeful!' Serena laughed.

'Other experiments,' I went on, 'have taken place in East Germany under the supervision of Professor G. W. Helse. His patients had all complained of reduced sexual desire, pain in connection with orgasm, difficulties with urination, and in many cases impotence. The Professor said recently: "Most of the patients under my care now have a greater sex drive, they no longer suffer impotence and other sexual disturbances; in fact, all are again enjoying a normal sex-life." '

'Which pollen do you suggest?' Serena asked.

'Cernelle of Vegeholme, in Sweden, produces a pollen product called "Politabs",' I answered. 'Doctors in Britain have found this most effective in combating chronic infections and inflammations where antibodies and sulfa drugs have proved ineffective. And Cernelle products are widely used for sex difficulties.'

'I've heard they have done a great deal of research in Sweden,' Serena said.

'Yes, Gosta Carlsson, who founded Cernelle, was the pioneer in this field,' I answered, 'and built the word's first pollen collecting machine in 1952.'

'How fascinating,' Serena cried.

'And to continue our train of thought,' I went on, 'Professor C. W. Heise has reported from Denmark that his male patients are enjoying a happier sex life after treatment with pollen extract. Incidentally, in Sweden alone more than 4,000 doctors are prescribing Cernelle pure pollen extracts to their patients.'

'Do you take it?' Serena asked.

'It gives me energy,' I replied, 'but I do find that pollen is inclined to make one put on weight. And there is one thing I would like to add.'

'What is that?' Serena asked.

'Just a word of caution,' I answered. 'Pollen is a live substance – one should always use it carefully at first. Some people are allergic to quite unexpected things and I do advise taking pollen in a very small quantity to start with, and when using pollen cream to test it first on the inside of the arm.'

'That seems common-sense,' Serena smiled.

'Pollen does help memory,' I continued. 'It is now considered a treatment for prostatitis, it increases one's resistance to harmful bacteria and combats infection. It is also believed to contain life's secret in its cell nucleus, but use it sparingly to begin with and watch the effects on yourself.'

'Anything else to do with pollen?' Serena asked.

'One which comes from Vienna is called Melbrosia for Men.'

'What does it do?' Serena asked.

'It is specially for men,' I answered, 'And once again it is flower pollen from specially selected flowers and Royal Jelly.'

'And it makes them virile?' Serena inquired.

'It does quite a lot of things,' I answered. 'It has been found in a series of clinical trials to be a great help to diabetics. Doctors worked on this for a long time before they discovered the excellent results with Melbrosia for Men on the growth of stunted children.'

'That's surely unusual?' Serena cried.

'It's very difficult to discover something to build up strength and increase weight in children,' I answered, 'but Melbrosia for Men has also been found to be useful in increasing the red corpuscles and the haemoglobin content of the bloodstream, so the two go together.'

'Why is it particularly good for sex?' Serena asked.

'Clinical tests carried out by Dr. Rudolf Frey, Head Physician of Korneuburg Hospital in Austria,' I told her, 'found that many patients showed a marked improvement after taking Melbrosia for Men in everything to do with memory, concentration, lassitude, exhaustion, and mental depression.

'All these things, of course, are part of the breakdown in sexual virility, and men who have taken Melbrosia for Men have reported the most excellent results in bringing back their vigour and their virility after only a short course of treatment.'

'How do they take it?' Serena asked.

'In capsule form,' I answered. 'One Melbrosia for Men is put under the tongue, preferably before breakfast. The result is fantastic, a man finds himself stronger, mentally, physically and sexually, within a few days.'

'Up to what age do they work?' Serena asked.

'Up to 100 if you like,' I replied. 'Dr. Urban himself is over sixty, and yet he can run like a young man of thirty. I've given them to even older men, and one friend of nearly seventy has just been married again to a young woman.'

'Surely he,' Serena said, 'wanted something very stimulating at that age?'

'Fortunately Dr. Urban has two things which are what we might call rejuvenating or sex pills which are remarkably effective in healthy people.

'The first is a rejuvenating elixir called Florapoll for both men and women. It contains the active substances of certain rare species of flower pollen, and those who have tried Florapoll said that not only do exhaustion and depression disappear within a few days of starting treatment, but there is a marked restoration of libido besides the remarkable results on the sex side. 'Florapoll incidentally has an excellent effect on patients with diabetes.'

'To return to the sex,' Serena said, 'are there any other products?'

'There is one called Melbrosia Executive, which is specially prepared for men suffering from so much stress and strain at their work that their wives have then taken lovers.

'Melbrosia Executive has had fabulous reports from Vienna and many Englishmen, whom one might call "Industrial Tycoons" have been very grateful for it.

'These Melbrosia products,' I went on, 'are made by a charming and exciting man, Dr. Paul Urban.'

'Why is he exciting?' Serena asked.

'He was a hero of the Resistance in Yugoslavia,' I replied. 'He was a most courageous Commander, and has remained a close friend of President Tito ever since.

'His great scientific knowledge has been of inestimable help to the Health Movement in this country.'

I shut up my notes at which I had been looking while I talked to her and rose from my desk.

'Is this all you have to say about love-making?' Serena inquired in surprise.

'The rest is up to the man and woman who want to love

and be loved,' I answered. 'Everyone is different, not only in body but in mind, personality and character. Everyone too has a personal secret.'

'What is that?' Serena asked.

'It is some little thing which for them excites passion more than anything else,' I replied. 'It may seem a quirk of the mind or rather of the imagination, but for each of us there is some special word, action, or thought, which sets desire alight.'

'Just as Honey has a potentiating effect on other products,' Serena suggested.

'Exactly,' I said, 'The match to the petrol tin! A man who is a good lover communicates his secret to the woman he loves, and the woman teaches him what excites her. It may be something very trivial like being kissed on the neck, but, to arouse her, it is all-important. Then, wanting only to give each other perfect happiness, together they find the full ecstasy of love.'

'A union of body and mind,' Serena said softly.

'Listen to the beautiful words a Hindu husband says to his wife when he consummates their marriage,' I begged her:

> ' "*United are our minds*
> *United are our hearts*
> *United our bodies*
> *I will bind thee with the bond of love*
> *And the bond shall be indissoluble.*" '

CHAPTER THREE

HONEY FOR HEALTH

'What about Honey for general health?' Serena asked.

'I was coming to that,' I replied, 'but I started with love and sex because there is nothing which more helps a person's health, both mentally and physically, than making love.'

'I have never heard anyone say that before,' Serena exclaimed.

'But, of course, it is common-sense,' I replied. 'If you are in love and your love is consummated, it both makes you happy emotionally and also stimulates physically your whole body. There is no other physical exercise which uses every muscle except the act of making love.'

'I think this ought to be said more often,' Serena declared.

'Of course it should,' I said. 'And people who say they are too old to make love when they are no more than middle-aged are really finished! It means that they have given up the last vestige of their youth and often, where a woman is concerned, the last vestige of her beauty.'

'Is it true that love really makes you beautiful?' Serena asked.

'My home,' I replied, 'was once rented by Dame Nellie Melba many years ago when she was quite an old woman. She went to Camfield Place for a holiday and when she was there she fell in love with a young man. Because she was in love her voice, which she thought she had lost, returned — that wonderful, fantastic voice which had thrilled the world. I always remember this story when I hear people saying

"I'm too old for that nonsense", or "I'm past that sort of thing".'

'Such idiotic remarks,' Serena agreed.

'I often tell people,' I went on, 'that if you no longer enjoy sex you are dead. You may be walking about doing things, but you are just a dead person because the spirit of life has gone. Sex is the Divine force which is poured through us all and it links us with the whole Universe.'

'I wish more people thought of sex like that,' Serena said.

'So do I,' I replied. 'But it is only the permissive society in which we live which has continued to make sex something scruffy and dirty or, as portrayed on the television, blatant and extremely ugly. It is, I admit, very difficult to portray the beauty of love and sex because it is indivisible. All these things belong to the spirit.

'Man in his search for God has always tried to capture beauty and portray it. Love, motivated by sex, has been responsible for some of the finest music in the world, the greatest pictures, the most moving poetry. Once we realize this, we shall stop sniggering. Love + sex is the Divine force in every one of us.'

'I agree with everything you say,' Serena exclaimed, 'But I do think that one's attitude to love and sex does depend tremendously on good health.'

'Of course it does,' I replied, 'and that is why I say over and over again that the most precious possession that anyone can have is their health. Think how terribly a lot of people abuse it!'

'Smoking, drinking, over-working!' Serena enumerated.

'And not eating the right food,' I finished.

'So we must put back into our bodies the vitamins which are destroyed by the way we live!' Serena cried triumphantly.

'You're learning!' I smiled. 'But of course that is right, and for good health I always start with vitamins. As I have said before, vitamins should be balanced, and it is a great mistake to take one vitamin alone. So the obvious solution is multi-vitamin tablets or capsules.'

'You think they are important to take with Honey?' Serena asked.

'I do,' I replied, 'and I will tell you about an amazing case where I am quite certain Honey with a multi-vitamin capsule triggered off a cure. There was an old woman living in my village who for twenty-five years had suffered from gangrenous ulcers on her legs. Two or three times a week the district nurse used to call and bandage her legs.'

'Horrible, painful things!' Serena exclaimed, 'and very difficult to cure.'

'I knew that the doctor had prescribed all sorts of different lotions to try to get rid of the ulcers,' I went on. 'Then one day I went to see the old lady. Her husband worked in the churchyard looking after the graves. I found they were both old-age pensioners and had just celebrated their diamond wedding; so you can imagine she wasn't very young.

' "I know you have trouble with your legs," I said to her, "and I wonder if you would like to try some vitamins. I'm sure they would help you and, anyway, alleviate some of the pain."

'She was only too willing to try anything, and I left her a pot of Honey together with some boxes of VM's, a multi-vitamin mineral capsule.'

'I am sure she was grateful!' Serena smiled.

'People are always grateful for health,' I said. 'When I gave VM's to Mrs. Indira Gandhi, Prime Minister of India, she told me that she had distributed what I had sent among her staff as well as taking them herself. It was a typically unselfish gesture that one finds so often in the East, and it meant all the more as it is so very hard to get natural vitamins in India.

'She told me later that her staff were all thrilled with the vitamins, and they all felt so much better on them! So I told my old lady with the gangrenous ulcers that she was in good company in taking VM's.'

'What happened?' Serena asked.

'Well, I suppose I left her enough to last about a month or maybe six weeks,' I said. 'Anyway, a little while later I said to our District Nurse:

' "Oh, by the way, how is the poor old dear with the gangrenous ulcers?"

' "Oh, I don't go there any more," she answered.

' "Not go there?" I questioned. "She isn't dead, is she?"

' "Oh, no," Nurse replied, "but her legs have been completely cured. Isn't it amazing after twenty-five years!'

'Well, I went at once to see what had happened, and the old lady told me:

' "I've taken nothing except your pills and the Honey. My husband and I both enjoyed the Honey enormously. We have never bought it before, I don't know why, and it certainly must be this and the pills which have cleared up my legs." '

'How extraordinary!' Serena said. 'I don't suppose anyone will believe that story.'

'I hope they will,' I replied, 'because it is the truth. And I'll tell you another story which is true, and which is hard to believe. My son and I went to Scotland last September, and our first guest was a very old friend who was, at one time, the tallest man but one in the British Army.'

'How tall is he?' Serena asked.

'He is 6 feet 7 inches,' I replied, 'and he was topped by only one other officer who was 6 feet $7\frac{1}{2}$ inches. When he arrived to stay he was limping, and I looked at him in consternation.'

' "What is the matter?" I asked.

' "I've got arthritis," he replied, "it's very painful and it's making me limp. I've been to the doctor, and I'm going to have treatment for it as soon as I go South again. But I didn't want it to prevent my coming up here, so I'm afraid you'll have to put up with me as I am."

'Well, my heart sank because there were only two things to do in Scotland in September. One was to fish, and the river was dead low, and the other was to shoot, which meant a lot of hard walking.

' "I'm afraid you're going to have rather a dull time," I said. "It is almost impossible to catch a salmon, and you will find the walking rather difficult."

'Having been a soldier he was prepared to put a brave face on it.

' "I'll start up the hill," he said, "and if I get too tired I shall have to come back."

'He arrived on a Sunday, and on Monday morning I looked to see what vitamins I could spare him. I gave him what I could spare from those I had brought up for my son and myself – there wasn't time to send South for more!'

'What did you give him?' Serena asked curiously.

'I gave him two Gev-E-Tabs – my own favourite multi-vitamin tablet – and four Bone Meal. Of course, there was Honey for breakfast and for tea.'

'What happened?' Serena asked impatiently.

'Well, believe it or not, having had vitamins and Honey on Monday and Tuesday, he said to me on Wednesday morning:

' "It seems like a miracle, but I'm not limping, and what's more I haven't got any pain." '

'It isn't possible,' Serena scoffed.

'It is true,' I answered, 'But unfortunately I didn't know then about an even more marvellous product to cure rheumatism and arthritis – Calcium Pantothenate Acid.'

'What is that?' Serena asked, 'I do not think I have heard of it before.'

'A lack of Pantothenate Acid results in fatigue, listlessness, digestive disturbances, headaches, irritability, heavinesss, mental depression, quarrelsomeness and recurring respiratory infections.

'I found that after months of pain, Calcium Pantothenate, which is derived from Pantothenic Acid, removes the pain and stiffness of arthritis.'

'Tell me about it from the beginning,' Serena begged.

'I have always believed, as I have said so often, that there is a natural Nature's cure for everything from which we suffer,' I began, 'but arthritis has been one of the most difficult!

'In the past few years Arthritis and Rheumatism have increased dramatically without there being any really effective products to cure or even relieve the misery and distress it brings to so many people.

'Arthritis has been suffered by human beings and animals since the beginning of time. Some years ago, while they were widening a new road on part of my husband's land in Scotland, the bulldozers unearthed the grave of a Chieftain's daughter who had been buried in the pre-Viking days. Although she had been quite young when she died, the doctors found signs of arthritis on the bones of her skeleton.

'I started what has been a terrible saga of pain and discomfort in February 1974 when I fell down in the Taj Mahal by moonlight. Everyone laughs when I tell that that was what happened, but actually from my point of view it was a disaster.

'The gateway to the Taj Mahal has a very high step and the Indians shone their torches on our faces instead of on our feet. I caught my toe on the step and fell forward, making my leg bleed very badly.

'But what I did not realize at the time was that I had put out the base of my spine. This pressed on the sciatic nerve and in a month's time I was in agony.

'I then started a long trek of trying to find someone to help me.

'I went to six osteopaths and had traction, I had acupuncture, I had injections! I took dozens of different so-called cures for rheumatism, arthritis, sciatica and gout!

'None of which really helped, and the only suggestion I had from doctors was that I should have the surgical operation which meant cutting off the end of the spine. This I was determined not to do!

'I was really getting desperate. I got to the stage when I could not walk more than a few yards, and it was very painful to turn over in bed. In fact I had to pull my legs round with both hands.

'Then a friend told me that she had seen on a television programme an amazing man called MacManaway talking to Ludovic Kennedy. It was said that he could do marvels with bad backs. Because I had nothing to lose I wrote to Major

MacManaway at the B.B.C. and asked if he ever came to London, as I understood he lived in Scotland.

'He rang up and gave me an appointment and I actually had no idea he was a Healer until I arrived at his mother's flat and met the most charming and delightful old lady of eighty who told me she had been a Healer for thirty years.

' "I worked very hard, but I never took money for what I did to help people," she told me. "But my son has a wife and three children and, as he has left the Army to continue his work, he has to charge a small fee.'

'It was in fact a very small fee, but as soon as I met Major MacManaway I felt that he had very special powers. I learnt later that he had discovered his power of healing in 1940 and later, with his wife, founded the Westlake Healing and Teaching Centre.

'To my great relief I did not have to undress, I merely sat in front of him and he put his hands on my spine and with a very small movement put the "tail" which was out of place into its proper position.

' "Now I am going to put on the heat," he said.

'I could feel waves of heat going up my back which vibrated all over my body. It was only when he had finished did I realize it was only his hands which had produced the heat!

'From that moment my spine was in the correct place but I had terrible adhesions of arthritis from the eighteen months in which I had been incapacitated.

'Then one day I was thinking about the problem and I read Adelle Davis's book which is now available in this country, called "Let's Get Well".

'I read that for arthritis she recommended Calcium Pantothenate which was a new way of taking Pantothenic Acid.

'She says in her book that deficiencies in this vitamin produce fatigue, listlessness, digestive disturbances, headaches, irritability, heaviness, mental depression, quarrelsomeness and recurring respiratory infections. She also said that Calcium Pantothenate removed the pain and stiffness of arthritis.

'This is something I had never heard of before, so I rang round the Health Movement to find where I could get it. I talked with Mr. Roger Lane, who told me he had some Calcium Pantothenate capsules which were not then on the market, but he said, "you must take it in large doses."

'He sent me his tablets which were 25 mg. each. This meant that I had to take four, three times a day. Almost immediately the pains in my leg and ankle felt better and it was easier to walk.

'I then found I could get the tablets in 500 mg, from the Cantassium Company. I talked to Dr. Robert Woodward who makes them and he told me that E. C. Barton-Wright, D.Sc., had been working on Calcium Pantothenate for some years with the most fantastic results!

'Of course we had not been told about it because doctors will never advertise their findings.

'Within a few days of taking four of the 500 mg. tablets of Calcium Pantothenate a day the pain was disappearing so quickly that I could hardly believe it! But I learnt that it was possible to obtain injections, which Barton-Wright and Dr. W. A. Elliott had also been using for a long time.

'I prefer injections and it only meant having three the first two weeks, two the third week and one the fourth week! But for people who find it difficult to get a nurse, the 500 mg. tablets are miraculous and it only means taking four a day.

'The latest scientific findings are that arthritis comes from a deficiency of Pantothenic Acid. Osteoarthritis in dogs, especially among pedigree animals, has been increasing during the last ten to fifteen years and is probably due to these animals being fed on highly processed canned foods.

'Pigs fed on a pantothenic acid deficient diet become extremely thin and emaciated and have a rough coat with loss of hair. They also develop what has come to be called "goose-stepping gait" in their hind legs which is due to osteoarthritis in their leg joints.

Barton-Wright and Dr. Elliott achieved the most remarkable results with vegetarian arthritics. When they were injected with a mixture of Royal Jelly and Calcium Pantothenate, they all showed a rapid disappearance of symptoms in fourteen days with remarkable increase in the blood Pantothenic acid level.

'Another doctor has said that if pregnant women were given a daily supply of 50 mg. of Pantothenate Acid they would not only prevent a miscarriage but their children would be born strong and that many of the ills, physical and mental, from which the human race suffers would be things of the past.

'Arthritis, whether rheumatoid or osteoarthritis, is on the increase the world over and there is no doubt that it is due to the world population eating more and more of the highly preserved foods which we in the Health Movement are well aware are dangerous.

'It is an insidious disease and may take many years before visible symptoms appear. We are all of us eating some Pantothenate Acid in our diet, inadequate though these amounts may be, but anyone who feels any twinges of pain – which means practically everyone in this country – from rheumatism, gout or any other allied disease, would be wise to take immediately at least 25 mg. of Pantothenate Acid a day.'

'What vitamins are really important to health?' Serena asked.

'Well, first of all, Vitamin E is the life, youth, and sex vitamin,' I replied, 'and that is why I think it is so essential to the human body.'

'What does it do?' Serena inquired.

'Well, first of all, it improves the circulation,' I answered. 'I am sure that one main reason why people become ill is that something has gone wrong with their circulation. Vitamin E helps to maintain a high level of oxygen in the blood, and we all know that oxygen helps to nourish the body's tissues, maintains the body's reproductive powers, and rejuvenates many other processes which would otherwise decline and degenerate.'

'I can see both youth and sex in that statement,' Serena smiled.

'Moreover,' I went on, 'I always suggest it to people who have varicose veins.'

'Will it cure them?' Serena inquired.

'I have a friend who was going to have her third operation on her legs,' I replied. 'She had actually booked her room in the hospital when I persuaded her to try Vitamin E in large doses. Last week she showed me her legs. There was only one tiny vein still visible, the rest had all disappeared.'

'That's amazing,' Serena cried, 'How many vitamins did she take?'

'She took six a day, in other words 600 units,' I answered. 'Dr. Shute himself – he was the real discoverer of Vitamin E – has told me that he doesn't really think that Vitamin E works in minimum doses. He believes it should be given in large doses continuously to get the right effect.

'For people who want to have babies it is essential,' I continued. 'A little while ago someone came to me in deep distress, who had been married for twelve years without having a child. I gave her a number of vitamins, but the most important among them was Vitamin E. Now they have a daughter whom they have called Barbara.'

'They must have been thrilled,' Serena said.

'They were,' I answered. 'And another friend was nine years without a baby, and after both she and her husband – I always insist on them both taking it — had taken Vitamin E, plus, of course, a foundation vitamin and various others which I consider important, they started a family and now have three children.'

'It seems to work for everything,' Serena laughed.

'It certainly does,' I replied. 'For people who think it's just for dizziness, hot flushes, and all those other tiresome symptoms which used to be part of the menopause, and now need not be endured any longer with Hormone Replacement Treatment.'

'What do you mean by that?' Serena asked.'

'You haven't heard of Hormone Replacement Treatment?' I inquired.

'No,' Serena replied.

'Then listen carefully,' I told her. 'Women can remain looking young and feeling full of vitality and energy for ever if they take oestrogen. This natural substance in the shape of PREMARIN prevents the change of life and all symptoms of it.

Eighty per cent of American women have Hormone Replacement Therapy, which means one in four do not suffer from hot flushes, night sweats, backache, headache, menopause depression, or the drying up or shrinking of the vagina which for some women can make intercourse painful. Oestrogen also prevents brittle bones in older women. A world expert on osteoporosis says:

' "A fracture has never been seen once the Therapy has been properly instituted."

'After an hysterectomy it is essential as it keeps a woman unwithered inside, prevents wrinkles and all the irritation, nerves and frustration of encroaching age.

'I take Premarin 1.25, a natural oestrogen, and I feel marvellous. A smaller dose is 0.65. I find most of the big Specialists and Gynaecologists are prescribing this today for women "in the change" and for the rest of their lives.

'Premarin is obtainable on the National Health on a Doctor's prescription. Ask him to read "The Lancet" page 135, 16th January, 1971, where it shows evidence from four important gynaecologists that oestrogen *prevents* cancer, especially the incidence of uterine cancer.

'I take, as advised, one Premarin tablet a day for three weeks, stop a week, and then start again. If my breasts feel tender or prick slightly, it means I have enough oestrogen in my body and I stop the tablets for two or three days. I think it essential to take Vitamin E with Premarin, but at different times of the day, i.e. Premarin in the morning and Vitamin E in the evening.

'There are three natural hormones, which are Premarin, Harmogen and Progynova. Insist on having one of these from your local doctor or see one of the many Specialists who now prescribe it.

'A book which tells you about all the research on this

exciting new treatment is "No Change" by Wendy Cooper, published by Hutchinson.

'Incidentally,' I added, 'Vitamin E is used in treating diseases of the eye.'

'I thought it was Vitamin A and B2 which affected the eyes,' Serena said.

'They are important, and for the average person they are enough to keep their eyes strong and healthy,' I replied, 'but if someone is starting a cataract or has inflammation of the retina, then Vitamin E is really effective.'

'What else does it do?' Serena asked curiously.

'It can prevent hardening of the arteries,' I replied, 'and blood blots in the veins, which we know as thrombosis or phlebitis, and this is all part of its wonderful effect on the circulation. But as far as you and I are concerned, what is so exciting is that it does retard old age.'

'Does it really do that?' Serena asked.

'They have proved it on animals, and now Dr. Aloys Tappel, a biochemist at the University of California, has said that in his opinion Vitamin E can slow down the ageing process in humans. "Ageing," he says, "is due to the process of oxidation, and since Vitamin E is a natural anti-oxidant, it could be used to counteract this process in the body." '

'Now how old do you have to be before you take Vitamin E?' Serena inquired.

'You can start when you are very young if you want to,' I replied. 'A lot of young athletes have found that it gives them tremendous strength and endurance. One boy I know was very distressed because he didn't grow.'

'There is nothing more miserable than being under-size when you are young,' Serena said.

'Or at any age if it comes to that,' I replied. 'Well, this boy was fourteen and he minded very much being smaller than the other boys of his age. I gave him four Vitamin E every day, and he shot up!'

'How delighted he must have been!' Serena said.

'He was indeed,' I agreed. 'It also made him feel so well that now he goes on taking it. There is really no reason why everyone shouldn't benefit from this wonderful vitamin.'

'Is it good for rheumatism?' Serena asked.

'There was a woman whose hands and arms were completely fixed with arthritis,' I answered. 'Her husband, who was a car-hire driver, came to see me in great distress. I suggested various things for her, the most important in my mind being Vitamin E. All this woman had been able to do was to sit in her chair all day, unable to move. After about three weeks her husband arrived one evening, with the tears running down his face. Her fingers had started to move.'

'How amazing!' Serena exclaimed.

'It was,' I answered, 'and after that she did the housework and the cooking. She had days when she still felt rather bad, but she got better.

'That was some years ago, today I should have suggested as well large doses of Calcium Pantothenate and the injections.'

'What about all these tonics which are for sale in the Health Stores?' Serena asked. 'Do you advocate them?'

'Of course, most of them are excellent,' I answered, 'and however many vitamins you take, you often need a little more. They naturally have vitamins in them.'

'Which one should one take?' Serena asked.

'Let me tell you something most exciting,' I suggested.

'Oh, do!' Serena cried. 'Why is it so exciting?'

'For a long time,' I began, 'scientists have thought that somewhere in the world there are precious vegetables, fruits, and herbs which are not available in the ordinary diet, but which contain health ingredients that could be of inestimable value to the human race.'

'I can understand that,' Serena murmured.

'The first discovery was the Acerola berry in Puerto Rico,' I went on. 'It was found to contain more Vitamin C than anything else in Nature, and what is so fascinating is that Acerola will not grow anywhere else except in Puerto Rico.'

'Why not?' Serena asked.

'No one knows,' I replied. 'Only in Puerto Rico does one

have the right complex of soil, sun, humidity, and so on for Nature to produce this natural Vitamin C miracle.'

'And then . . .?' Serena questioned.

'The search for QUINTESSEN began,' I replied.

'Is that what it is called?' Serena asked.

'It describes something very, very special,' I smiled, 'a collection of plants, herbs, and fruit so precious that they have come from every part of the globe. Some have been recognized and respected by native populations for centuries and become part of their diet. Some have never been used before.'

'Is Quintessen a medicine?' Serena asked.

'No,' I replied, 'nor is it principally a vitamin ingredient. It is a complex of natural food factors from ingedients we have not until now included in our daily diet. It is something extra, extra *special*.'

'I do think that sounds exciting,' Serena cried.

'It is,' I agreed. 'The essential essences of sixty rare substances drawn together from the most remote corners of the earth can now be enjoyed by you and I in our homes.'

'Do tell me more,' Serena begged.

'Well, Quintessen, which has over a hundred active ingredients, is divided into five major parts,' I answered, 'which are:

1. Exotic Tropical Fruits.

2. Rare Indigenous Herbs and herbal extracts of reputed activity.

3. A selection of Sprouted Seeds wherein the living seed germ is extracted by an enzymatic process.

4. Biochemic Tissue Salts are included to ensure mineral balance.

5. An elixir prepared from extracted Kelp, Rose Hips, Acerola Cherry, Molasses, Mount Hymettus Honey, and citrus fruits known for their valuable vitamin content.'

'It sounds fabulous!' Serena cried.

'It is,' I agreed, 'and just listen what fruits are included –

54

Mango, Bael, Paw Paw (which I love), Guava (Pandit Nehru gave me the first one I ever tasted), Passion Fruit (the most exotic taste in the world), Hearts of Palm, Ugli Fruit (I ate this in Mexico), Grenadilla, Arbutus, Avocado (which is wonderful for the skin), Kumquats, Plantain, Lychees (which are simply delicious), and with these is an edible vine leaf from Greece, and lots of other tropical fruits.'

'My mouth is watering,' Serena laughed, 'tell me more.'

'I can't tell you about all sixty of the herbs,' I laughed, 'but here are a few:

1. *Dioscorea* – this is a wild yam indigenous to Mexico and is considered to be one of the most important plants ever discovered. Its extracts are employed to overcome sterility (in both the male and the female) and impotence, and it will tone up the whole system by its wonderful effect on the glandular system.

2. *Ginseng* – the Chinese ascribe wonderful medicinal virtues to it, and have used it for thousands of years. In its early days Ginseng root was so valuable that it was the property only of the Chinese Emperor. The sick take Ginseng for its curative properties, while the healthy use it to resist disease and make themselves stronger. Men over forty use Ginseng to preserve their virile powers and to avoid the so-called male climacteric. It is common to find in China men taking Ginseng who procreate children at the age of eighty and more.

3. *Hydrocotyle Asiatica Minor* – is also called Fo-ti-Tieng. This herb has a reputation of being one of the finest of all herbal tonics. It possesses great life-sustaining properties, and those who take it live to a great age. It has attracted scientific research in many European countries of recent date, and a French Professor who studied the herb has claimed to have found in it an unknown vitamin which he terms Vitamin X. This vitamin appears to have a marvellous rejuvenating effect on the brain cells and endocrine glands.

4. *Damiana* – is largely prescribed on account of its aphrodisiac qualities. There is no doubt that it has an enormous

beneficial action on the reproductive organs, and it also acts as a tonic to the nervous system.

5. *Kava Kava* – this herb was first scientifically described by a father and son team of Botanists who accompanied Captain Cook on his second voyage in 1776. They were given a coconut shell filled with a strange liquid. At first it tasted pungent and rather soapy, but next came a fresh feeling in the mouth lasting several hours. A small quantity made everyone relaxed and friendly. it is suggested that a wine glass can produce within a short time a profound dreamless sleep with no morning-after effects. Unlike alcohol the herb does not impair mental alertness.'

'What a wonderful group of magical Herbs!' Serena exclaimed, as I paused for breath.

'It is wonderful,' I agreed. 'Quintessen includes Stimulant herbs, Tonic herbs, Alterative herbs, Nourishing herbs, Soothing herbs, and Nervinc herbs, in fact Quintessen is the magic wand to glowing, exciting health.'

'I see there is Honey in this wonderful preparation,' Serena said.

'Of course there is,' I replied, 'because Honey will trigger off all those wonderfully rare but explosive treasures which have been kept secret for centuries.'

'Which Honey did you say was used?' Serena inquired.

'Hymettus Honey from Olympus in Greece, the seat of the Gods,' I told her, 'and I believe Quintessen will give us some of that glowing, radiant, almost spiritual health which the ancient Greeks believed was their heritage from the Gods.'

'Tell me about some more tonics,' Serena commanded. 'What about Bio-Strath, I know that is a big seller?'

'I introduced Bio-Strath to England in 1964,' I answered. 'Last year nearly a million bottles were sold in this country.'

'I hope you've got shares in it,' Serena laughed.

'That is what everyone says,' I replied, 'and the answer is NO. I don't own shares or have a financial interest in anything to do with Health because I must be impartial. Also I try everything I recommend and refuse to endorse anything which does not suit me or my family, which is why so many people trust my judgment.'

'And you knew Bio-Strath was a winner as soon as you tasted it?' Serena asked.

'It helped me,' I replied simply, 'so I wanted it to help other people. It was, of course, the first of the herbs "digested" in yeast to come to this country. I've written the story in *I Search for Rainbows*, and the fact that it has helped a lot of people is only too obvious by the sales.'

'It's obvious it must be good!' Serena agreed.

'It is good,' I replied, 'but in this thrilling new science of nutrition we are always discovering something new. Nothing stands still. Isn't it extraordinary to think that vitamins themselves have only been discovered in the last fifty years or so, and some of them – Vitamin E for instance – have only recently been found to be essential for human health.'

'What a lot we've learnt!' Serena said.

'I have!' I replied. 'I nearly died in 1950, and vitamins saved my life. That is why I became so interested in them.'

'How did you know that you should take vitamins?' Serena asked.

'I had heard a little about them in America,' I replied, 'but my doctor had during the war been a prisoner in Singapore. He knew the terrible death roll of our men working on the Burma Road was principally due to beri-beri – or lack of Vitamin B. So he gave me lots of vitamins and I recovered!'

'Were there natural vitamins in those days?'

'No,' I replied. 'People are so lucky today because they can get the whole range of natural vitamins grown by Nature. But do remember that Natural Vitamins are only found in Health Food Stores, the ones in chemist shops are artificial.'

'Made with chemicals,' Serena added.

'Of course,' I agreed. 'That is why I say keep to vitamins and elixirs, like Gev-E-Tabs, Quintessen and Bio-Strath, which we know contain all the precious natural vitamins, including many, I am sure, which have not yet been discovered.'

'What do you mean by that?' Serena asked.

'When you take a natural vitamin supplement,' I replied, 'wholly derived from natural products and brought together from all parts of the world, as in the case of Quintessen, you get the bonus of these extra nutrients which science hasn't yet succeeded in duplicating.'

'That's exciting,' Serena agreed. 'What about single vitamins?'

'Add them to your Gev-E-Tab team,' I replied. 'Again make sure they are natural. Once again I must remind you, Serena, that you can't take too many *natural* vitamins. They are only food, and if you take more than your body needs, they are eliminated in exactly the same way as a big meal or that extra helping.'

'But I'm sure it's better to take too many vitamins than too few,' Serena laughed.

'Of course,' I said, 'how sensible you are getting about this.'

'Vitamin C is important, isn't it?' Serena asked.

'Tremendously important,' I answered. 'And as you know I don't approve of citrus fruit: oranges and grapefruit are far too strong for the average person's stomach, besides often causing them to have a bad complexion.'

'I always thought fruit was good for the complexion,' Serena interjected.

'If you really want to see bad complexions,' I answered, 'look at those belonging to American and Canadian women who are always screaming for their orange juice first thing in the morning. If I take orange juice it brings me out in spots, and if my children take it, it brings them out in eczema. The best possible source of Vitamin C is rose hips prepared carefully to preserve the vital Vitamin C and blackcurrant juice.'

'There is one thing I want to ask you about,' Serena said, 'and that is Royal Jelly. We have heard so much about it over the years and I've always wondered if it's as effective as the advertisements claim.'

'I think it is good,' I answered, 'and for some people it really works. In fact they feel amazingly better as soon as they begin to take Royal Jelly. As you know, it comes from the

Queen Bee, who is literally stuffed with Royal Jelly. She swims in a considerable excess of food, all of an extraordinarily rich composition, and it is this food which ensures that the Queen lives four to five years, while the life of an average bee isn't more than forty-five days in a working period.'

'I should have thought that was definitely a class distinction,' Serena remarked dryly.

'It is, but at the same time they work her very hard,' I smiled. 'She becomes a real production machine capable of laying over 2,000 eggs a day, and two million eggs during her life.'

'Well, if her food can be taken by us,' Serena said, 'it ought to do us good.'

'There have been a great many fantastic claims made about Royal Jelly,' I said. 'Scientists believe that it acts as a stimulant in the human body and that the body is invigorated so that physical and intellectual capacity is improved. They also say that it can help to cure tuberculosis, entero-colitis, anaemia, and depression. Dr. Telatin of the psychiatric Hospital of Imola in Italy has found Royal Jelly mixed with pure Honey is marvellous for neurosis.

'Another Specialist says: "Royal Jelly causes an improvement in fertility, especially when diminished by age, and stimulates the sexual activity when its diminution takes its roots in a mental disturbance, such as the simple fear of impotence."

'Royal Jelly is also an amazing source of Pantothenate Acid.'

'Is there anything else I should try?' Serena inquired.

'There is something else,' I went on. 'I've thought for some time you have looked rather tired and exhausted, and I think, like so many women, you are without knowing it suffering from an iron deficiency.'

'I think I've always needed iron,' Serena agreed, 'but it's difficult to take and sometimes upsets my tummy.'

'That is something this new, exciting iron tonic I am going to give you won't do!' I told her. 'Called Floradix, it has just been introduced into this country, and I find it simply fabulous. It does something for which I've been looking for a long time – it gives one an almost instant lift.'

'That's what I want now,' Serena groaned.

'In a number of scientific studies in Southern Germany,' I said, 'the doctors found that almost every other woman, and one girl in two, suffered from a hidden iron deficiency.'

'What are the symptoms?' Serena asked.

'General fatigue, a tendency to headaches, grooves in the finger-nails, excessive susceptibility to infection, particularly colds, are the most usual signs,' I replied.

'Why should we be short of iron?' Serena inquired.

'First, modern food is deficient in iron, so we do not obtain enough with our meals and do not absorb what is there. Then we lose iron in so many ways.'

'What are they?' Serena asked curiously.

'A woman loses 10–50 mg. of iron with her normal period,' I answered. 'This amount should under ordinary circumstances be replaced by her food within a period of four weeks, but if her food, as is now universal, is lacking in iron content, then she soon develops a dangerous iron deficiency.'

'I know one loses iron when having a baby,' Serena said.

'The iron demand of the child in the womb, the blood loss during delivery, and the iron required during nursing, results in an iron loss of 600–1,000 mg.,' I told her.

'Do children require iron?' Serena asked.

'Of course,' I replied. 'Children and adolescents require an increased amount of iron for their haemoglobin and the growth of their body cells. New-born babies only have an iron reserve of approximately 36 mg., which is quickly used up for the foundation of new cells, and it is most important to remember that during the first year of their life the blood volume is tripled.'

'How interesting!' Serena exclaimed. 'I had no idea of that.'

'Breast milk,' I went on, 'contains only a very little iron and cow milk practically none. So you can see how many children become very anaemic during the first years of their life. As cultured iron yeast is used in this product the iron is very easily absorbed, and it also contains Vitamin C and B complex.'

'What else is there in it?' Serena asked.

'A herb extract and real Honey as well as glucose,' I answered. 'It suits young and old as well as people in-between like yourself. What is more, it is delicious to take and everyone I have given it to looks forward to their dessert-spoonful three times a day.'

'It is a liquid form then,' Serena said.

'I like it best as a liquid,' I replied, 'but there is also a tablet for those who want to take it in the office or who are taking part in outdoor sports.'

'Is it good for athletics?' Serena inquired.

'The tablets were used with great effect in the German Himalaya Expedition of 1966,' I answered, 'the Munich Hindukusch Exploration Trip in 1967, and in 1968 in Mexico City the German Kanu Olympic Team, who did very well, all took Floradix.'

'What about the women?' Serena asked.

'Inge Schell took it,' I replied, 'and she is convinced it helped her to become the woman World Champion of the Year.'

'Floradix must be wonderful!' Serena exclaimed.

'It is,' I agreed, 'and the Olympic team said positively that it is "an invigorating agent". That is what interests me. You and I need invigorating in our busy lives and this is something which doesn't like so many tonics, lift you up and drop you down. It really builds up one's body, making it stronger, younger, and more enduring.'

'Floradix for me!' Serena cried. 'You'll be surprised how much I can do in a week or two, and, of course, I'll take extra Honey as well. Do I also need a laxative?'

'Honey, of course, possesses natural laxative properties,' I said, 'so it's excellent for children who are often constipated, and it thus helps to create wonderful complexions. There is nothing more dangerous to health, or to the complexion, than not going regularly to the lavatory. I am appalled how many people think that it doesn't matter if you miss a day. After twelve hours the poison in our bowels begins to seep all over the body, so you can imagine that anyone who isn't regular is bound not only to have bad breath, but also a sallow, spotty complexion, and often endless headaches.'

'How much Honey should I take at night?' Serena asked.

'I take it with cider,' I said, 'but if I need what my mother called "a dose", I drink Culpepers' Aperient tea, also vinegar with Honey.'

'How do you make them?' Serena asked.

'In an ordinary teapot,' I replied, 'or Heath and Heather supply little muslin bags containing exactly the right amount. Pour boiling water on it in the ordinary way, and let it stand for about ten minutes. Pour it into a cup and add a tablespoonful of Honey. Stir it well and drink it. I will guarantee you will go to sleep in front of *Peyton Place*, or whatever your favourite television programme is, so it is best to take it at the very last minute when you are actually in bed.'

'It sounds just what I need!' Serena exclaimed.

'What is so wonderful,' I went on, 'Is that the healing quality of Honey can then go on working all night, and you will find that you wake up in the morning feeling not only bright and ready for a day's work, but happy, and with none of that "Oh, no, not another day" attitude which many people have after a night of disturbed sleep or after taking sleeping-tablets.'

'I shall certainly try it,' Serena said, 'and I do think sleep is important, don't you?'

'It is important for everyone,' I answered. 'Do remember that children get terribly tired. I have always let my children sleep as late as they like at week-ends. So many people stick to a routine seven days a week, and this contributes to the tension which is really a major illness these days.'

'You think it's a good thing to break the habit, say, of waking at 7.30 or 8 o'clock?' Serena asked.

'I think people need to have their sleep out at least twice a week,' I said, 'and there is no reason why, except for babies who have to be given a bottle, people shouldn't sleep late on Saturdays and Sundays.'

'What about breakfast?' Serena asked.

'A friend of mine, who has a big family, doesn't worry with breakfast on Sundays,' I replied. 'When they are awake they go downstairs and help themselves if they are hungry. She always has something like cold ham if they don't want to cook anything, or there are plenty of eggs. Very often the menfolk sleep right through until lunch-time, and that is why I think as a family they are so healthy and well; it is very seldom that any of them miss a day's work.'

'It is certainly an idea,' Serena said doubtfully, 'but men always seem to want to play games or watch them on Saturdays.'

'They can still sleep a little later than usual,' I answered. 'This mad rush at week-ends, when one is working terribly hard in the week, is a tremendous strain on one's physical endurance. Have a break whenever it's possible, and when you go on holiday do allow yourself to rest at least part of the time.'

'I am sure you're right,' Serena said.

'There is only one thing I want to add,' I went on. 'I am convinced that Honey is the greatest and most wonderful preservative of youth, because Honey in itself never grows old.'

'What do you mean by that?' Serena asked.

'Honey improves with age,' I replied, 'it's the one food product that does. They have never yet found any Honey that was too old to be edible. A few years ago Honey was found in a tomb in Egypt, which was known to be over 3,000 years old. It was in a perfect state of preservation, and delicious to eat.'

'How amazing,' Serena said.

'There is no doubt that the Ancient Greeks regarded Honey as an Elixir of Youth. The philosophers of Athens believed that the life span could be doubled if they could

63

discover the right combination of foods, and for them Honey was the most important food of all.'

'Did they live to be very old?' Serena asked.

'Apollonius lived until he was 115, and he was supposed to have eaten Honey every day,' I said. 'We can, of course, compare this with the great age of the people in Bulgaria today, who we are told eat the scrapings off the bottom of the hive, and think nothing of being over 150.'

'I believe people in Poland also live to a very great age,' Serena said. 'Wasn't there a king who was a bee-keeper?'

'There was indeed,' I replied. 'Piast was the king you are talking about, and he lived until he was 124. But these figures really mean nothing: there are exceptional examples in every country all over the world, and I am not really concerned with anyone living to be very, very old, unless they are also feeling very, very young.'

'Nobody wants to be old and doddery,' Serena murmured.

'What I am certain of is that Honey possesses some magic quality which can help us to feel young, so that old age is never troublesome,' I continued. 'As you say, it doesn't matter being old in years, but it does matter being decrepit. Blind, deaf, and a burden on everyone, that is what we wish to avoid; and I do believe that Honey, if taken every day, can help us to feel, look, and be young, whatever our birth certificate says.'

CHAPTER FOUR

HONEY FOR HEALING

'Tell me about Honey for healing,' Serena asked. 'People are always saying that it is wonderful, but I've never heard of any doctor prescribing it.'

'Not modern doctors,' I replied, 'but in Ancient times the physicians believed it to be an unfailing healer for almost every type of ailment, and they were possibly right!'

'What about today?' Serena inquired.

'Well, we are just beginning to return to the old ideas. It is rather the same as when you were a child – you thought your parents were all wrong, and then when you get older you begin to see that mother did know best,' I smiled. 'Only this time it's a thousand great-grandmothers and great-grand-fathers who used Honey and were immeasurably streng-thened and healed by it.'

'How did you learn about Honey?' Serena asked.

'Well, I think the first time I really thought about it,' I replied, 'was when I read a story about a man who had a petrol filling station in the Arizona desert. It was miles from anywhere, but he and his wife made a living from the trucks and the occasional travellers who passed by. One day some-thing went wrong and the gasolene tank blew up, and in trying to put the fires out the owner was most terribly burnt.'

'It sounds terrifying!' Serena exclaimed.

'Fire always is,' I replied, 'and many more dangerous fires happen every year than we ever hear about. To continue with my story, the man's whole body was badly burnt and there was no medicament in the house which they could use to alleviate the terrible pain. Fortunately they had only that very day taken the Honey from their hives, so the wife and the mother of the burnt man covered him in Honey, and wrapping him with gauze like a cocoon, they put him in a car and rattled him fifteen miles over dusty, bumpy roads to the nearest hospital.'

'It must have been a nightmare journey,' Serena said sympathetically.

'It would have been,' I replied, 'if the man had been in the agony he had suffered when he was first burnt; but from the moment they applied the Honey he suffered no pain.'

'I don't believe it,' Serena ejaculated.

'It's true,' I declared, 'and, what is more, the burns healed without leaving any scar on his body. It was this that made the doctors begin to think and realize, as their forerunners thousands of years earlier had realized, that Honey can be an invariable healer.'

'So they rediscovered Honey!' Serena smiled.

'They found that the germ that causes dysentery dies within forty-eight hours and that the chronic bronchopneumonia germs die on the fourth day, and the germ that causes typhoid – and may cause peritonitis – on the fifth day. All these die in far quicker time than could be achieved by penicillin or any other antibiotic.'

'Is this proved by scientists?' Serena asked.

'The figures I have just given you come from the United States Bureau of Entomology in Washington,' I said. 'But in this country our hospitals also are beginning to appreciate the value of Honey.'

'I think that's wonderful,' Serena said. 'What else does Honey cure?'

'Well, I think the most important development in the last few years,' I replied, 'is that it is found to be a splendid heart stimulant. The late Sir Arbuthnot Lane, who was an old friend of mine, and whom I admired enormously, was almost the first person in the medical faculty of Great Britain to use Honey as a heart and muscle stimulant, and he was an outstanding specialist of his day on stomach ailments.'

'I must tell my aunt at once,' Serena said, 'she has a weak heart and we are always worrying that she will do too much.'

'Do tell her about Honey,' I said. 'And Honey is marvellous for older people because it fights anaemia. Honey helps to maintain the right balance in our blood, and this, of course, is tremendously important as you get old. So many people say that their blood "is getting thin".

'Dr. Arnold Lorand, who wrote an excellent book called *Old Age Deferred* says:

' "As the best food for the heart I recommend Honey. Honey is easily digested and assimilated, and it's the best sweet food as it does not cause flatulence and can prevent it to a certain extent, promoting the activity of the bowels." '

'That is certainly excellent advice for old people,' Serena agreed.

'I've had a lot to do with the elderly,' I answered, 'and I know that they crave sugar. It absolutely astounds me that in our Old People's Homes all over the country we never insist that the food they are given contributes to their good health. They eat white bread, white sugar, lots of starchy pudding, and no one ever seems to demand that they should have Honey, whole-meal bread, and, although it's expensive, plenty of protein in the shape of meat.'

'But would they like Honey in their tea?' Serena asked with a smile.

'Of course they would!' I asserted. 'Haven't you ever tried Honey in tea? To begin with, it is almost impossible to tell the difference in flavouring between Honey and white sugar, and secondly Honey is sweeter. Moreover, Honey at night makes old people sleep.

'My mother is always complaining that I never told her this, and she had to wait to hear me saying it on the radio. But, however she learnt it, she now takes Honey in hot water or hot milk every night when she goes to bed. It really helps her to sleep. As she is ninety-eight, like other old people she doesn't sleep for very long, but the sleep she does have is deep and restful, owing to the fact that she has taken her Honey.'

'I had heard that Honey in hot water was good for sore throats,' Serena said.

'Some people swear,' I replied, 'that a gargle made with a cider vinegar, to which Honey has been added, removes a sore throat immediately.'

'Would it help a cough?' Serena asked. 'My daughter Sally always gets a cough in the winter.'

'Honey and lemon juice will help a cough,' I replied, 'And if you like to add a few drops of glycerine, I think it makes it even more soothing. But Sally wouldn't have a cough at all if you gave her Honey all the year round. I've already told you that I cured my husband's bronchitis by seeing that he had comb-honey night and morning every day of the year.'

'I really shall have to do what you tell me,' Serena said. 'I've been trying to make a note of all the things we've talked about, and very soon I shall be able to write a book on it.'

'In about 400 B.C.,' I went on, 'the great doctor Hippocrates, whom you must have heard of, recommended Honey as a means of curing ulcers. And now, only a little while ago, a doctor writing in the *Middlesex Hospital Journal* stated that Honey applied to external ulcerated or infected surfaces had a definite bactericidal power.

'A leading British gynaecologist five years ago startled the medical world when he said he found Honey, in dealing with wounds and infected conditions, far superior to any drugs.

'The Senior Consultant Gynaecologist and Obstetrician, from the Norfolk and Norwich Hospital, Dr. A. P. Bentall, said that he always used honey for open wounds, just as his predecessor, Dr. Michael W. Bulman, had done, who had written a most interesting article on the subject.'

'I can't think why we haven't known about all this before,' Serena complained.

'That's what Eamonn Andrews said to me,' I replied, 'when I was on his clever *Tonight* programme and we were talking about the magic of Honey. You know, when it's something so ordinary as Honey, people turn a blind eye or a deaf ear to what they see or hear, and it just doesn't sink in.

But once you have tried things the results are tremendously impressive.

'I had a letter from a woman the other day who told me that I had recommended a pure Honey Cream to her for her face.

'Well, apparently she had a very deep wound in her arm that had been troubling her for some months. The doctor's tried almost everything on it, and it wouldn't heal. Because I had been so effusive about the Honey Cream for removing spots and blemishes from her complexion, she put the cream on her arm also.

' "You won't believe it," she wrote, "I hardly credit it myself, but in one week, after all these months of trial and failure, the wound has healed." '

'What is this Honey Cream?' Serena asked.

'It is just called Pure Honey Cream, made by Mrs. Conway in her home. It is completely pure and a wonderful aid to beauty,' I answered.

'The two seem synonymous,' Serena smiled.

'What else does Honey heal?' Serena asked.

'Almost everything!' I claimed. 'My mother's housekeeper had a gathered finger and you know how painful that is! When my mother told me about it on the telephone, I told her to suggest Honey. Her housekeeper covered her finger in Honey, wrapped it in a bandage, and it was cured in twenty-four hours!'

'I had a gathered toe for two months,' Serena moaned, 'and I had to have antibiotics!'

'I expect you know,' I went on, 'that in Ancient Egypt, China, and all over the East, Honey was used for embalming.'

'I had heard of that,' Serena agreed.

'Apparently they still use it in Burma,' I continued. 'And of course in the East they use Honey as a preservative in cakes, sweet-meats, everything you're offered to eat in an Indian household. This is because Honey preserves food in a climate where everything decomposes very rapidly.'

'How delicious they are – but so fattening!' Serena sighed.

'Another of the things Honey does,' I said, 'is to strengthen the bladder. I have found it extremely effective with old people, and for years it has been used to prevent bed-wetting among nervous children. With them Honey has a double effect: firstly it acts as a sedative to the child's nervous system; secondly it attracts and holds fluid and spares the kidneys, with the result that a child does not wet the bed at night.'

'How much does one give a child?' Serena inquired.

'About one teaspoonful of Honey last thing,' I answered, 'And old people can take more. As I've already suggested, Honey in hot water or hot milk will not only make them sleep, but prevent them having to rise so often in the early hours – one of the most tiresome aspects of getting old!'

'What about migraine and hay fever?' Serena asked.

'I think that Honey can be wonderful for migraine,' I answered. 'I had a woman write to me only a little while ago about her husband's migraine, and she was almost in despair! He had given up his business and retired quite early in life because he had migraine once or twice a week, and he just couldn't go on. Well, I gave him a diet of protein, no milk, which I think is very important, no white sugar, and no bread.'

'No bread!' Serena ejaculated.

'No bread,' I said firmly. 'Anything stodgy is extremely bad for migraine, sinus, and catarrh. Then I suggested that he should take lots of Honey, vitamins, especially Vitamin A and Propolis. In the last six months he has had only one attack, and that, I suspect, is because he let up on his diet. Now he is planning to go back to work and take up his old job again.'

'That is amazing,' Serena declared. 'And does it work in the same way for allergies?'

'Allergies seem to be cured, or possibly prevented by Honey,' I replied, 'And one of the best things for people with allergies is to chew a square inch of Honey-Comb Cappings for about five minutes. They should treat it as though it was chewing-gum and go on chewing until there is very little left, then swallow it. The Propolis or bee-glue of the Honey-comb is of tremendous value to people who are subject to allergic reactions in the breathing tract. Of course, as Dr. Jarvis says in *Folk Medicine*, they must eat Honey as well.'

'Why are the Honey-combs so good?' Serena asked.

'No one has yet discovered the active principle in Honey-comb,' I answered. 'It's another part of Honey magic. All we know is that the combination of Honey and Comb-Honey produces wonderful results.'

'I've been told that children who are brought up on Comb-Honey until they are sixteen never have colds, hay fever, or nerve disorders,' Serena said. 'Is that true?'

'I am sure it is; I have found it wonderful for asthmatic people,' I answered. 'I remember a little girl with terrible catarrh who could hardly breathe at all. I suggested Honey-Comb Cappings and her mother told me that after chewing them she rushed at her crying: "I can smell you, oh it's lovely! lovely!" '

'How did this happen?' Serena inquired.

'I asked a doctor,' I replied, 'and he told me that the Honey-Comb Cappings for some unknown reason shrink the nose tissues and improve the condition of the Mucous Membrane.'

'I shall try it next time I have a stuffy cold,' Serena vowed.

'Chew Honey-Comb Cappings every hour for four to six hours,' I told her, 'but personally I think that Propolis is even more effective.'

'What is Propolis?' Serena answered. 'I do not think you have mentioned it before.'

'In Austria they have rediscovered a honey product which, to me, is extremely exciting. Propolis, a name which stems from the Ancient Greek and means "a system of defence" was used by the Assyrians to heal wounds, inflamed eyes and tumours.

'The Egyptians recognized its efficacy in embalming their dead. It had been forgotten since 400 B.C., when it was prescribed by the Greeks in the treatment of abscesses and open wounds. Theophrastos, a celebrated philosopher in 390 B.C. gives exact instructions on how and where this resin may be found.

'It is, in fact, collected by the bees and is a yellow-golden viscous substance which closes the fissures of the hive and prevents any bacteria entering into the "Holy of Holies" where the queen lives.

'Dr. Paul Urban has had very stringent clinical tests done on Propolis and has found it to be the most effective natural antibiotic that has ever been discovered!

'Doctors took into the Public Hospital in Klosterneuburg 250 people suffering from stomach ulcers, colitis and severe gastric conditions, and they were treated with Propolis. Two hundred and forty-four were completely healed within a fortnight.

'After another test in the Ear, Nose and Throat Clinic at Lujubljana, Professor Kern spoke with great enthusiasm of the effect of Propolis on patients with inflammation of the throat and oral cavities. The patients chewed the Propolis lozenges, which are so delicious that I have great difficulty in keeping them away from my grandchildren who like them as sweets.

'In as little as six to ten hours after commencement of the treatment with the Propolis Bonbons, almost all the patients were free of fever; they felt no pain when swallowing and their general condition was very much improved.

'The doctors' findings are, I think, extremely interesting. In fifteen acute cases, especially in the case of children, they found an improvement had taken place after only a few hours.

'In the case of patients suffering from chronic inflammation of the oral cavity and gums, the symptoms of the inflammation were hardly noticeable the following day.

'Another test, made by Frau Dr. Edith Lauda, is one of the most interesting that I have read for a very long time. What the doctor wished to establish was whether Propolis had an anti-bacterial effect on the human skin.

'Fifty-nine patients with really bad acne, from which they

had been suffering for several years, were treated with the Propolis ointment which is now obtainable here.

'One patient had been treated unsuccessfully for thirty years by a great number of dermatologists and clinics, and yet after two Propolis treatments the skin was free of inflammation and only very small marks of the acne were visible.

'Almost equally spectacular was the case of the patient aged forty who tried every possible treatment for the acne which covered her whole face, and in two weeks the acne completely disappeared after treating herself at home with the Propolis tincture and the ointment!

'Twenty-five cases of acne simplex were completely healed at home within a week.

'This is thrilling news for those teenagers and older women who write to me in despair about their complexions, many of whom have got to the stage where they feel they cannot go out because they are so embarrassed by the appearance of their skin.

'To me it proves that there are many more things in natural medicine which have either not yet been discovered or, more interesting still, have been forgotten over the centuries.'

'It all gets back to honey,' Serena smiled. 'When would you give a baby honey?'

'First of all in its bottle,' I answered. 'Doctors who have studied the effect of Honey added to the diet of infants, have found that Honey does not cause diarrhoea, which so many other items in a child's diet are inclined to do. Of course as a child gets older Honey is a tremendous help when they are cutting their teeth. The sedative effect of Honey then is invaluable.'

'I think it's very exciting!' Serena exclaimed, 'when you find that something as simple as Honey will not only prevent diseases and heal them, but will also make people strong and healthy from childhood.'

'And good too,' I added. 'Honey has always been connected with religion. The bow-string of the Indian Love

God Kama is formed by a chain of bees, and many of the Yogis used Honey as a special religious food, believing it had the power to cleanse and revitalize.

'I am sure that people who take a lot of Honey become kinder and nicer and more loving. Perhaps everyone who is very healthy should be like that, but I think it is particularly true of Honey eaters. I am convinced in my own mind that while Honey cures and energizes the body, it also inspires the brain and warms the heart.

'It's a lovely idea!' Serena smiled.

'We all need much more warmth, friendliness, love, and understanding,' I continued, 'if we are ever to lead this world out of war and chaos into peace and plenty. The Israelites knew what they were talking about when they went to look for a land which "flowed with milk and Honey".'

CHAPTER FIVE

HONEY FOR BEAUTY

'How do you think I look?' Serena asked, coming into the room in a very pretty pale blue dress, and turning round to show herself.

'I think you look wonderful,' I declared.

'Don't you think I'm a little thinner?' she asked, 'and look at my complexion.'

'It's certainly very clear,' I answered.

'It's transparently clear,' Serena corrected, 'and I've been working on it as a surprise for you. What do you think I've been using?'

'I can guess,' I answered. 'Honey!'

'Yes, of course,' she laughed, 'and I've been taking it. And do you know, I not only feel marvellous, but I am so much better tempered. Peter remarked on it today and suggested I must be having a secret love-affair; he'd never known me in such good spirits!'

'What did you tell him?' I asked.

'I told him,' Serena answered, 'that I had fallen in love with him all over again. He was absolutely delighted and went off to the office purring like a cat who has got at the cream.'

'You are becoming quite a clever person,' I said.

'No, I am just a Honey-eater,' Serena answered. 'If they all feel as I do, the Marriage Guidance Council will be able to put up their shutters.'

'Well, your complexion is certainly glowing proof that Honey taken internally as well as externally does work,' I said. 'And now I've got something really exciting to tell you on the health front, which you won't need now, but you'll be delighted to have to take in a few years' time.'

'What is it?' Serena asked. 'And if it's for someone who is getting on in years, I've got a message for you from my eldest sister. You know that Helga is fifteen years older than I am? Well, I've been telling her on the telephone all the things we were discussing, and she's asked me if there is anything you can give her. She says she is getting old, dull, and flabby, and she is really ashamed to come to London from the country because not only has she got nothing to wear, but anything she puts on looks awful.'

'I don't believe a word of it,' I said, 'Helga is almost as pretty as you, Serena.'

'She used to be lovely,' Serena admitted, 'but she has rather let herself go. She has four children, which I suppose pulls you down a bit, and she didn't do exercises or anything after they were born. Quite frankly her figure is a mess. It's rather tragic because her husband is so good-looking and I am always frightened that he will be snatched away by some scintillating blonde in a bikini. You know what women are like when there's an attractive man about: they don't worry if he is married, they just try to get their claws into him!'

'Tell Helga not to worry,' I said. 'I've got the very thing she needs, and this is what I was going to tell you about.'

'What's it called?' Serena asked.

'You remember I talked to you a little while ago, when we were discussing energy, about a product from Vienna called Melbrosia.'

'Yes, of course I remember,' Serena said. 'You said it was particularly good for giving people new energy. I think you said it contained Royal Jelly.'

'That's right,' I said. 'You are a good pupil to remember. Well, Dr. Paul Urban and his team of Scientists working in the Melbrosin laboratories have discovered that certain pollens which they use in their products are better than others for women.'

'How extraordinary,' Serena said. 'It must have taken a lot of research to discover that.'

'Apparently they've been working on this idea for years,' I said, 'And now they have found that they can produce a really remarkable effect with certain selected pollens, when they are combined with Royal Jelly, in restoring a woman's youthful appearance and her figure.

'I can't wait to tell Helga,' Serena said.

'They have called this product Melbrosia PLD,' I said.

'What does PLD stand for?' Serena interrupted.

'*Pour les dames,*' I replied, 'in other words, "for the women". They say that it normalizes, restores, and improves, both psychologically and physically. I think that is very important for women like your sister, who are beginning to feel depressed and dull, and think they must give up.'

'You're right,' Serena agreed, 'and a lot of the trouble is because they just give up trying.'

'Melbrosia PLD gives them a new enjoyment of life, a new energy, and new vitality,' I went on. 'Now you may think that that is exactly what I said the ordinary Melbrosia would do, but this new product has a very special difference.'

'What is that?' Serena asked.

'Well, first of all,' I explained, 'the skin becomes tighter, and the tissues of the body become firmer, the whole effect being that a woman looks much more youthful. But most important of all, the muscles of the breasts are strengthened and lifted.'

'I don't believe it,' Serena cried.

'It's true,' I answered. 'They experimented on an enormous number of women, and in practically every case of women under fifty, the effect on the breasts has been fantastic. Over fifty, and even over sixty, they have had a large amount of success, but they cannot promise a 100 per cent result at that age.'

'It's certainly very exciting,' Serena said, 'how does one take it?'

'Melbrosia PLD comes in rather attractive red capsules,' I

said. 'The normal dose is one capsule each day, taken fifteen minutes before a meal, and on an empty stomach. They ask you to put the capsule under your tongue and keep it there for a few minutes so that the majority of the important substances it contains can be absorbed by the mucous membrane of the mouth. This is quite usual with medicines which have to be absorbed before they reach the stomach.'

'How long does one take it before there are any results?' Serena asked.

'The first result with most woman is that nails grow long and hard,' I said, 'although Dr. Urban tells me he did not anticipate this. He says the course should be continued without interruption for thirty days, and if it is a severe case of saggy body, then there is no harm in taking up to three capsules a day, one before each main meal. In fact, of course, there is absolutely nothing in Melbrosia PLD that can hurt one, however much one takes.'

'Does it really work?' Serena inquired.

'I have already seen amazing results on women to whom I have given it,' I answered her. 'I am quite convinced that pollen has various different properties, and that, by breaking it up into different categories for different conditions, the researchers are on the verge of something very exciting and very new.'

'I must certainly tell Helga about this,' Serena said. 'What else can you suggest?'

'I think she would be wise to take Vitamin E, at the same time,' I answered, 'Because Vitamin E, as I have already said, is so tremendously important in promoting circulation.'

'And, while we are speaking of beauty,' I went on, 'you know the habit which is most destructive to women – smoking. Any woman who smokes has a yellow skin by the time she is forty. I've yet to find an exception. Whenever I see a woman with a beautiful pink and white skin, I know she does not smoke.'

'Do you really think it makes people ugly?' Serena laughed.

'I think there are three things which destroy beauty in

women,' I replied, 'and the first is smoking. To begin with there is nothing feminine about smoking. It makes a woman smell, and it's an established fact that tobacco on a woman has a very different and much nastier smell than on a man. I don't know why, it must have something to do with the pigment of the skin; but if you are close to a woman who smokes a lot, you will find she really does smell extremely unpleasant.'

'I have noticed that,' Serena agreed.

'And the sad thing is they have no idea of it,' I went on. 'A young girl came to my house the other day and she chain-smoked. She left cigarette ends with lipstick on them all over the house. She threw them about in the garden and, apart from all this untidiness, I really didn't like sitting near to her because she smelt so unpleasant. And when I told her so, she was absolutely astonished!'

' "I don't smell," ' she said angrily.

' "Of course you do," I answered. "When I open a letter, I know immediately if the writer smokes. As I don't smoke myself, I am very sensitive to smell. So you can imagine what it's like for me to have to sit next to someone who smokes as much as you do. It really is very unpleasant."

'Poor girl, she was quite shattered but it was a lesson she had to learn sooner or later.'

'I can't think why girls want to smoke when so few young men do nowadays,' Serena said.

'I feel exactly the same,' I answered. 'Some young men were saying the other day that they really disliked kissing a girl who smoked because it left a taste like vinegar on their lips!'

'With most of them it's just a stupid habit,' Serena stated.

'And a very dangerous one,' I added. 'Did you see the statistics which were published the other day about mothers who smoke while pregnant?'

'No, I didn't see them,' Serena replied, 'What were they?'

'A doctor who had studied a large number of pregnant women,' I answered, 'found that on the average there is one miscarriage in every twenty-four births, but with mothers who smoke the risk is one in thirteen. Besides this, it is known that where a mother has smoked during pregnancy, the child is smaller, weaker, and more prone to disease.'

'That is terrifying,' Serena cried.

'It's wicked,' I declared. 'Anyone who can prejudice, for their own selfish enjoyment, the future life and health of an unborn child is really evil.'

'Yet I'm afraid women will go on smoking,' Serena said.

'They are stupid enough to think they can give it up any moment they want to,' I said, 'but like everything else it requires will power. And usually when the moment comes they can't. But anyone who smokes, if they care about themselves, their health, and their looks, must take Honey.'

'Why?' Serena asked. 'No! Wait! I know the answer! Honey is a healer.'

'Of course,' I approved. 'Smoking is so stupid, so wrong, because it affects the respiratory tract, and if we cease to breathe we die. So, that is a very important part of the body to us. Therefore the respiratory tract, which gets red and inflamed and, of course, discoloured with nicotine when we smoke, can be helped to a certain extent and kept from very serious damage shielded by Honey.

'But there's something worse than that which smoking does, which is that it inhibits oxygen from the heart. That is why when people first stop smoking they get fat. The oxygen surges over their bodies, and they feel extremely well and extremely hungry. So they eat too much to start with and put on weight.'

'Then they become hysterical and start smoking again,' Serena cried.

'But if only they would persevere,' I replied, 'and not go back to smoking, then gradually the body would balance itself and they would reach their proper weight.'

'But will they be as thin as they were before?' Serena asked.

'They will be breathing,' I answered. 'I had a man in my employ who went to the doctor last winter with bronchitis, and do you know what the doctor said to him? He said:

"Either you give up smoking or else in two years' time you won't be coming here to see me because you'll be dead!" That man was under forty.'

'Why did he smoke so much?'

'It was just a habit he had got into,' I replied, 'increasing until he was buying forty or fifty cigarettes a day. And he was a working man with six children! So apart from anything else, it was a senseless, idiotic extravagance.'

'Which he couldn't give up,' Serena murmured.

'Or rather he wouldn't,' I suggested. 'Another man I knew had very bad varicose veins. He wouldn't admit they were due to smoking, but when he was taken into hospital to be operated on, they wouldn't allow him any cigarettes. When he came out I didn't recognize him. He had gone in thin and extremely bad tempered; he came out a chubby, red-cheeked, jolly little man, with no varicose veins, and full of laughter and good spirits!'

'And what happened after that?' Serena asked.

'He has gone back to smoking,' I answered, 'and he has another very bad varicose vein, which will, in a few months' time, take him back into hospital again.'

'It seems crazy!!'

'It is,' I agreed, 'and the latest figures in smoking are:

1. Lung Cancer is twice as common as all the other cancers put together.

2. Smoking increases the age of smoker's blood by forty years.

3. Dr. Calder in the Lancet says that tobacco smoke destroys Vitamin C in other people who are not smoking.

4. A baby from a mother who smokes during pregnancy is smaller, lighter and more prone to disease.'

'What are the other two things which you think destroy beauty in women?' Serena sked.

'One is alcohol in excess,' I replied. 'The worst drink where a woman is concerned is gin, but any alcohol does harm because it destroys the vitamins in our bodies! Therefore if you drink, drink only a little, and put back into your bodies the vitamins which have been taken out.'

'Which are?' Serena prompted.

'Vitamin B and Vitamin C,' I said. 'The best thing when one has had a certain amount of drink at a dinner party is to take four B-Compleat tablets and four Bone Meal when you go to bed. In the morning, as soon as you wake, take a table-spoon of Honey, and several tablets of Vitamin C. You certainly won't feel any ill effects, and if you don't drink too often you won't see any.'

'And the other thing?' Serena asked.

'Sleeping-tablets,' I replied. 'They are guaranteed to make a woman ugly quicker than anything else I know. They relax the face, accentuate the lines, and take away the colour. However young a woman may be in years she will look old in the morning after taking sleeping-tablets.'

'The doctors hand them out quite freely,' Serena pointed out.

'They don't care how you look,' I replied. 'After all, who does care except oneself? Don't be such a fool as to take any form of sleeping-tablet or tranquillizer. They not only destroy one sooner or later, but they destroy any vestige of prettiness one may ever have had very, very quickly.'

'Why should they be so damaging?' Serena asked.

'Let me put it to you very simply,' I said. 'They slow down the brain to enable you to go to sleep. Now, as we have said so often, the body works as a balanced whole. Therefore you are not only slowing down your brain, you're slowing your whole body.

'This makes you more prone to disease, and it takes a lot of the elasticity of youth. We have already shown that you can get a relaxation from tension by taking Honey. But Honey in itself is a natural sedative, while anything stronger is not only wrong but really dangerous.'

'What do you mean by that?' Serena asked.

'A friend of mine,' I replied, 'a man, always took a sleep-ing draught every night. I never realized this, but I always thought he was rather vague and had difficulty in following what was being said in the conversation around him. I used to think it was due to his being slightly deaf, but I know now it was because he didn't really connect with what was happening, owing to the effect of his nightly sleeping-capsules.'

'I've noticed that my uncle, who takes them, sometimes fluffs his words,' Serena said reflectively.

'It's a sure sign,' I said.

'I do see it is frightening,' Serena admitted. 'We are now a nation of pill-takers.'

'I know women who get up in the morning in the new town of Hatfield,' I said, 'where you would think they had everything that was desirable in their new houses on their new estates, with their new shops and their new schools – and they take two aspirins first thing to help them through the day.'

'What for?' Serena exclaimed. 'It's crazy!'

'Yes, of course it is,' I agreed, 'and what is more, too much aspirin can send you bald.'

'Does it really?' Serena asked apprehensively.

'A woman came up to me at a meeting the other day,' I went on, 'and she said: "Do tell me what I can do about my hair. It's getting thinner and thinner, and there never was very much of it!"

' "Do you take aspirin?" I asked, quite out of the blue because I had just been reading about it.

' "As a matter of fact I do," she answered. "I take a lot of aspirin."

' "Then there's every likelihood of your becoming bald," I warned her. She was simply horrified, and I don't think she'll take aspirin in future!'

'In some diseases aspirin is necessary,' Serena demurred.

'If a doctor prescribes it, then of course it must be,' I answered. 'But I can't help feeling that there is very likely a natural cure which would be quite as good without the use of drugs. But then I'm prejudiced, I'm so frightened of all these drugs and tranquillizers; they have done such terrible things to my friends.

'A doctor who is working in a big London hospital told me last week that at least fifteen per cent, if not more, of the people occupying beds in that particular hospital were there because they were suffering from the side-effects of drugs they had taken to cure some other disease!'

'I have heard that the side-effects of drugs are increasing,' Serena said.

'Unfortunately it's true,' I answered. 'The drugs being manufactured today have side-effects which are not apparent when they are first put on the market, just like thalidomide. In fact, we get back to what I said in the beginning – never, if you can possibly help it, put anything that you know is an artificial chemical into your mouth, in either food, drink, or medicine.

'Of course, this is an impossible rule to keep strictly, but where you choose the natural and unprocessed food, then you are saving yourself from all sorts of unknown dangers.'

'And now tell me about Honey for the face,' Serena said.

'I thought we'd get to that sooner or later,' I laughed. 'First of all there is the most lovely face cream made with Honey and Beeswax. It is called Nectarene Skin Food. It is made at Holgates Honey Farm in Wales. I started to use it only a little while ago, but I was astonished at the difference it made to my skin.'

'But you always have had a good complexion!' Serena protested.

'I owe it to vitamins and Honey,' I laughed, 'but I promise you Nectarene Skin Food is something very special. The formula was evolved in 1957 to include the maximum quantity of Honey and Beeswax and yet avoid excessive stickiness.'

'Would it help someone who has had plastic surgery?' Serena asked.

'It is what I would use under similar conditions,' I answered, 'and I recommend Vitamin E oil, for anyone whose face has been burnt, wounded, or damaged in any way.'

'I must get some at once,' Serena said excitedly. 'What about pollen creams?'

'There are lots of pollen creams,' I replied. 'The best is Honey Pollen Cream, made by Ronald Hagman. It is used by a great number of actresses and people in the public eye, who have to keep their complexion clear and beautiful. A girl wrote to me this week saying: "It's marvellous! I'm so thrilled with my new face that I fear I may attract the bees!" '

'I've always heard that Cleopatra used Honey on her face,' Serena said.

'Many of the great beauties all through the Ages have used Honey,' I answered. 'You can do it yourself. Lie down and cover your face with Honey and you will find that it tightens the skin, at the same time giving it a fresh glow which is not obtainable with any other product. But it is sticky, and who has the time?

'You can't go to bed covered in Honey without getting it all over the pillows, and I can't imagine that your husband would find it very alluring! So we have to use it somehow in a form of cream, or a mask.'

'Is there a Honeymask?' Serena asked.

'There is indeed,' I replied, 'and it is made by Maria Hornes.'

'Oh, tell me about it!' Serena pleaded.

'It comes from Austria,' I replied, 'Where a famous skin-doctor experimented on peasant farmers. Now anyone who has seen the peasants working in Europe knows how old looking and wrinkled they become very early in life from exposure to all weathers. That is the reason why I always tell women to protect their skin against the elements.'

'I thought that fresh air was good for the skin,' Serena queried.

'I always remember Clare, the pretty Duchess of Sutherland, saying the same thing to me,' I replied. 'She and a friend of hers were walking about in Scotland unmade-up and with their faces turned towards the sky.

' "What are you doing?" I asked.

' "We are letting the fresh air get to our faces," Clare replied.

' "Have you seen what fresh air does to stone houses up here?" I asked. "You must be crazy! Always protect your skin."

'They were very surprised, and I went on to explain how the most beautiful and softest skin we have in our whole body is on the insides of our arms and between our legs, where it seldom sees the light of day.'

'Of course that's true,' Serena exclaimed, 'but I never thought about it before.'

'Always keep your face covered by a foundation cream,' I said. 'I use a heavy protective cream because I live in the country and am out in all weathers. Then I add Cyclax face powder, which is pure and contains a modicum of grease, so that it never moves or gets blown away. In fact, it's the ideal powder for the working girl. You can make up in the morning, and without worrying about your face you look exactly the same at six o'clock in the evening.'

'What a boon to career women!' Serena exclaimed.

'And many mothers,' I smiled.

'But to get back to the Honeymask, the doctor found that the peasants had aged prematurely from being always out in the blazing sun or the bitter cold. He felt that Honey could be the answer, and he invented a face-mask, which was based on Honey and a specially prepared vitamin formula.'

'What does it do?' Serena inquired.

'It is absorbed deep into the tissue cells,' I replied, 'and helps to activate the circulation, tone up the muscles, and bring into operation everything which is necessary for re-vitalizing the skin.

'When the doctor was carrying out these experiments, my friend, Maria Hornes, happened to be staying in the neighbourhood. She is a Hungarian, who knows an enormous amount about skin regeneration, because she herself had a terrible motor accident when she was young, and had great difficulty in bringing her face back to normal. She asked the doctor to show her the results of his experiments. She saw all the photographs, before and after the treatment, and she tells me the difference was simply amazing.'

'How long did the treatment take?' Serena questioned.

'Maria Hornes told me that some cases took several months if the patient was old and weather-beaten, but those between thirty and forty re-created a new texture to their skin in quite a reasonable time.'

'What is the mask made of?' Serena inquired.

'Marie Hornes found,' I replied, 'that the main ingredients in the doctor's treatment were Honey, the roots of plants which grow in the Alps, and five different vitamins, one of which is of course Vitamin E.

'I've seen the result of this mask, Serena, and tried it. By degrees it helps reduce the sagginess of the cheeks and neck, the swelling of the eyelids, the puffiness under the eyes, and gives a firmness to the contour of the face.'

'It sounds fabulous!' Serena cried.

'It is indeed,' I agreed. 'The skin seems to glow after one has used it, and one's complexion really does look young and blooming.'

'I can't wait to try it,' Serena said, 'or am I too young?'

'There are instructions for every age,' I answered. 'In the twenties, for instance, the doctor advises that a girl should use the Honey Face Mask once a fortnight for three months, and then once a month. But in the fifties and over, it should be applied every third day for two months and then weekly for three months, the treatment being reduced gradually to once or twice a month.'

'What is the mask called?' Serena asked.

'It's called FM29,' I replied. 'I can't think why nowadays all our Health products have to be numbered like motorcars, but it's the fashion, and I suppose we have to put up with it.'

'I think it's rather a good idea,' Serena said. 'I'm sure that we have got suspicious of things that have glowing titles, especially when we find they don't work.'

'I promise you this will work,' I answered, 'and it is far easier to apply than Cleopatra's.'

'What else can we use?' Serena asked.

'For everyone every day, I know nothing better than the Celaton Face Creams,' I replied. 'They all contain Honey, and I use Night Star Special at night and Day Moisture in the morning.'

'Do you suggest that for me?' Serena asked.

'No, because you are young. What you need is ordinary Night Star Face Cream and Day Moisture in the morning, but for any woman over fifty the Night Star Special has ingredients which definitely rejuvenate the skin.

'What I think will suit you is "Be Lovely". It is an exciting hand-made anti-wrinkle cream with honey and the special new ingredient collagen, which clinical tests have shown definitely removes wrinkles and lines.'

'How lovely! Where can I get it from?'

'It's made by Anna Chisholm and later I will give you her address.'

'Are there any more new creams?'

'Yes, a wonderful new and exciting cream called "Vitamin FF Cream". This is really rejuvenating and there are tablets, too, called FF/100 which gives you "New Youth".

'That is what I call it and it really is an answer to all our prayers.'

'What does it contain that is so special?' Serena inquired.

'It is the whole Vitamin F Complex and contains not only the ordinary Vitamin F but the rare natural form known as 6.9.12 Vitamin F. (Octadecatrienoic Acid).

'In the body, normal Vitamin F is converted very slowly into this rare form of Vitamin F, but as one gets older this process gets even slower. By providing the rare form of Vitamin F in the cream, we have by-passed the process that the body normally carries out. Now it provides the Vitamin in its readily assimilable form to build the intermediacs vital to life.'

'Where can I get it?' Serena asked excitedly.

'At the moment only from the Cantassium Company but I expect it soon will be in the Health Stores. It recreates our cells and makes us not only look lovely and young again but feel simply marvellous.'

'Anything else?' Serena asked.

'New creams are being invented every day,' I answered. 'By next month someone will have come up with another wonderful product, another new and exciting invention. That is why I always advise everyone who is interested in

Health to follow our research in the magazine, "Here's Health", and also to join the Health and Happiness Club.'*

'What is that?'

'It is a Club for people who live far from a Health Store, have children who make it difficult for them to get out and also do not know what to buy.'

'It sounds very useful.'

'It is. Everything recommended by the Club has been tried by me personally or by my family, and I write explaining exactly what the products do.'

'How helpful.'

'It saves people from buying the wrong things and the Club also sends its members samples of new and exciting products all for £1 a year.'

'There is a lot going on in the Health Movement,' Serena said.

'Yes, Health manufacturers from all over the world are exchanging their knowledge, their research, and their products,' I answered. 'In this way the sky's the limit for a new approach to health for everybody.'

* 25 High Street, Alton, Hampshire

CHAPTER SIX

HONEY FOR NERVES

'One of the most important diseases of modern living,' I said to Serena, 'is "nerves".'

'I expect it is,' she agreed, 'But when people say "it's my nerves" in a solemn voice I always want to giggle.'

'A great many people have got into the habit of putting everything down to nerves,' I said. 'Actually they are not far wrong, because the nervous system of the body is all-important, and we ignore it at our peril.'

'I suppose people think that nerves are independent of our other physical reactions,' Serena said reflectively.

'On the contrary,' I said, 'nerves are part of the chain reaction the emotions cause through our whole system. Actually there are three nervous systems which carry messages from our brain to the muscles and organs of our body.'

'What are they?' Serena asked.

'The one of which you are most aware is the one by which you talk, laugh, walk, and cry,' I replied. 'This is the central or voluntary system. It is this central nervous system which tells you when you are hungry, when you are cold, and, of course, when you are unhappy.

'The second system deals only with the organs of sense, that is to say those connected with seeing, smelling, hearing, feeling, and tasting.

'The third system – the autonomic system – is involved entirely with internal activity, and controls our muscles, veins, arteries, heart-beat, breathing, expansion and contraction of blood vessels, as well as the mechanism for digesting our food, storing it, and dispensing with all that is unnecessary.'

'Good gracious! It sounds like a computer!' Serena exclaimed.

'I think that is exactly what it is,' I replied, 'a human computer. But unfortunately we cannot command our nervous system to stop working, we cannot turn it off! It is vitally important to every one of us that the whole system, which reacts automatically to our emotions, should work harmoniously, and be in good health. Otherwise we can damage our nerves and have what people call a breakdown.'

'Then the question is,' Serena said, 'How do we keep our nerves in good condition?'

'We feed them,' I answered. 'The nerve cells of irritability are cells that are hungry, just as the nerve cell that is tired reacts because it needs food to keep it from becoming exhausted.'

'How much food is necessary to replenish the nerve cells and keep them well?' Serena asked.

'Specialists and doctors agree,' I replied, 'that nerve cells degenerate if they are made to expend their energy without 100 per cent replacement. This is why a balanced diet is absolutely essential for everyone who wishes to keep well, and the most dangerous thing people can do is to starve their body so as to get thin, and leave what old people quite wisely call "their nerves on edge".'

'Well, what then do we need?' Serena demanded.

'All the vitamins,' I replied. 'As the nervous system works over your body from the top of your head to the soles of your feet, you need every vitamin, and that is why it makes me so angry when people say, "Oh well, I'll just take one vitamin, and if it doesn't do me good I shall know you are talking nonsense". How can I give one vitamin to a person who has two eyes, ten fingers, ten toes, all sorts of complicated internal muscles, organs, veins, arteries, and thirty yards of intestine?'

Serena laughed.

'It sounds funny when you say it like that.'

'It's not funny,' I said, 'when you realize how people drive themselves into an acute depression and melancholia, and often into a state of lunacy or to the verge of suicide, simply because they harass the brain by starving their wretched unconsidered nerves.'

'I'm sure you are right,' Serena said.

'I'm quoting very much higher authority than myself,' I replied. 'Sir James Paggett, a British doctor who studied these things, said once: "You will find that fatigue has a larger share in the promotion and transmission of diseases than any other single causal condition you can name." '

'I suppose so many complaints can be attributed to nerves,' Serena said.

'Headaches, of course, migraine, and all mental illnesses,' I answered. 'Whenever I consider mental illness, I always think of a wonderful mental clinic there is in America, where, when a patient seeks admission, they insist that he or she must go first to an annexe and stay there for two months.'

'What happens there?' Serena asked.

'The patient is given proper food,' I replied, 'plus vitamins, and taught to relax. The clinic says that 50 per cent of those seeking admission go home completely cured.'

'It makes one wonder,' Serena said, 'whether we are feeding people right in our mental hospitals.'

'I wish I could say yes,' I answered. 'You know as well as I do that few people in this country have really studied the effects of food on disease, except a few nutritionists who are often dismissed as cranks.

'I have seen the food offered in many institutions and nursing homes which may be good and nourishing from an old-fashioned standpoint, but nothing is done to encourage people to eat the food that is really good for the nerves.

'Also I have never yet found a mental home where they were giving the patients natural vitamins. Synthetic vitamins perhaps, but never the natural ones.'

'And there is a great difference, isn't there?' Serena asked.

'There is one very obvious difference,' I replied. 'Synthetic vitamins are manufactured in factories, and they are made of chemicals; so, although they may help, you are still putting more chemicals into a body which is already overloaded with them.

'Natural vitamins are food. They are made from Rose Hip, Wheat Oil Germ, Brewers Yeast, herbs grown organically on ground that hasn't been polluted with pesticides. I contend therefore that it is impossible for natural vitamins not to do you good.'

'Can nerves cause diseases like arthritis?' Serena asked.

'Of course they can,' I replied. 'Neuritis and muscular ailments, heart disorders, and, of course, nearly all the disturbances of the gastro-intestinal tract, can all be symptoms of nerve cells that lack energy and want food.'

'Are you sure there isn't one particular vitamin which is important?' Serena asked.

'Neuritis can frequently occur when Vitamin B1 is inadequately supplied,' I answered, 'and this is the same vitamin which is particularly important to the brain. But once again I have found, as I have told you so often, that the vitamins themselves like a balance, and the Vitamin B's work best when they are combined together.

'But B1, thiamin, is particularly important for any brain work. They have done tests with it in hospitals by asking questions of patients when they were deficient in Vitamin B, and then asking the same sort of questions after Vitamin B had been injected into their bodies.

'In every case the ability to remember, clarity and quickness of thinking were quite extraordinary in the patients who even half an hour before had seemed almost morons.'

'I've always heard that Vitamin B1 was of tremendous importance,' Serena said.

'Nurses have done tests on themselves in hospitals,' I said. 'Without Vitamin B1 they found their work was much harder and they were far more exhausted after the long hours of being on duty. But once again I do beg people who want to take this very wonderful vitamin to take a foundation vitamin first, which will also, of course, include Vitamin B1.'

'What do you suggest then for nerves? Vitamins and lots of them?' Serena said.

'Vitamin B6 which is essential and really does magic away nerves, irritation and restlessness.'

I smiled as I added:

'It's also good for slimming.'

'Tell me about it quickly,' Serena ordered.

'I have always resisted every sort of pressure to advocate slimming treatments or to recommend any of the slimming products which are in the Health Movement as well as the Chemist shops,' I replied.

Quite frankly, I have always believed that they were dangerous and that slimming was something one should consider very, very carefully before one begins to diet.

First of all I usually ask the person who asks for my advice:

'Who are you slimming for? I have never yet met a man who did not like a handful!'

They laugh, but they still go on worrying about their attractive feminine curves which have been admired since the beginning of time and which make a woman look like a woman.

It becomes an obsession, their husbands run away with a plump blonde, their children find them irritable, hysterical and tearful, their neighbours hurry in opposite directions. But they still go on slimming!

We have to realize that everyone is different and that while some people are 'Pharaoh's lean kine' others are naturally well covered. Quite frankly, as I belong to the latter group, I think one is happier, more content and more vital when one has a little protection not only against the weather but against the stress of modern-day living.

When I had an operation three years ago, I lost two stone on the operating table and all my women friends came round afterwards crying:

'Darling, you are fashionable at last!'

'I am going to get fat again as quickly as I can,' I replied.

They despaired of me but although I was gracefully ethereal, my appearance would not have persuaded anyone to take one vitamin, let alone those which make us energetic, vivid and beautiful!

What would have happened to all of my Crusades? What is more, when you are over fifty and you start to slim you cannot keep a lovely face and have 36 inch hips! My advice, because one slims downwards, has always been to women to keep their beautiful faces and *sit down*!

But now at last I am breaking my golden rule of not writing about slimming, because from America has come a new and natural way to being slim of which I really can approve.

Mary Anne Crenshaw has discovered how to slim in an easy manner which is healthy, which does not deplete the body's natural substances and is not dangerous!

All it consists of is taking four important ingredients. They are all important to us all, and I have written about them very often, but we have not previously put them together!

These four thin friends are—Lecithin, Cider Vinegar, Kelp, and Vitamin B6.

First of all, because it is important, you must keep to your ordinary healthy diet which only means cutting out the unnecessary carbohydrates.

These are of course white bread, that poisonous white sugar, white flour and all the 'gooey' foods made with them which ruin the shape of a body over-night!

You can, as you well know, eat as much protein as you like, but while you are doing the diet do not consume a lot of fruit or drink an abnormal amount of alcohol. Both of these contain high amounts of carbohydrates.

We are so lucky, for now we actually have some capsules which contain Lecithin, Cider Vinegar, Kelp, and Vitamin B6. They are called Formula 3+6 Capsules. Take two or three after each meal and wait to take *in* your clothes.

If you are very overweight, to get down to what you want to be, I should also take at the same time extra amounts of these four natural substances. Let me explain why they are important.

This food is found in every single cell of the human body – thirty million of them – and its concentration in the brain is 17 per cent to 20 per cent. Lecithin is high in phosphorus and Linda Clark, one of the most important dieticians in the United States says:

'No phosphorus, no brains!'

But Lecithin does not stop at the brain; it is essential for the function of all glands, including the sex glands.

Lecithin raises both our mental and physical efficiency and speeds up the recovery-rate of nerve and muscle tissues subsequent to stress. It is particularly important to the nervous system which regulates and controls all the vital processes of the various organs in the body. Therefore people who talk about 'my nerves', who worry and quickly get lines on their face, require large doses of Lecithin.

Lecithin is of great importance for those also doing heavy physical labour or engaging in strenuous sports. During physical activities there sometimes comes a time when the body can no longer respond to the demands made upon it and the muscular system becomes exhausted. The more quickly the muscle recovers, the more effective an athlete can be and for this Lecithin is really important.

We have known this for a long time but a doctor in America found that when he was giving patients Lecithin, because it proved so effective against excess cholesterol, the patients not only felt better and could do more, they also lost weight! So here was the first indication that Lecithin could help those who were crying out to slim.

One can also buy Vita-Buerlecithin which is a delicious tonic.

'I have a friend who is suffering from a nervous tic,' Serena said. 'Would it be good for her?'

'It would be excellent,' I replied, 'and it will also help anyone with hardening of the arteries. For ordinary people like myself who are certainly not ill, after all the vitamins and things we take, Lecithin is what I need for my brain.

When I feel tired, after I've dictated perhaps 6,ooo words or I've motored for miles, made a speech, shaken hands with everyone present, and motored home again to find a mountain of work waiting for me, I take Vita-Buerlecithin.'

'Any time of the day?' Serena inquired.

'Any time of the day or night,' I answered. 'If I'm unable to sleep through worrying – of course we all worry at times over some problem or other – or I wake up and don't drop off again, I often take a spoonful of Vita-Buerlecithin, and then I sleep peacefully. After all, worry, insomnia, and tiredness are all things which can be traced back to those tiresome, troublesome nerves.'

'I must get a bottle at once,' Serena said.

'To return to our Four Slim Friends,' I went on.

CIDER VINEGAR

This is the second 'friend' and everyone has already said it is useful for slimming. I think it has helped enormously, especially when it is drunk at lunch and dinner instead of white wine or soft drinks which do put on weight. But Cider Vinegar plus Lecithin is something new and very important to remember.

KELP

Number three is Kelp. Again something I have talked about and taken for a long time and which I have always believed is particularly important to health. Kelp, because it is seaweed, has a great deal of iodine in it and iodine is something which burns up the surplus fat in our bodies.

Kelp is also wonderful for the skin and the hair and now I am convinced that it is Kelp which helps to make the body firm and young with the Lecithin and Cider Vinegar.

VITAMIN B6

This is the Vitamin about which I am wildly enthusiastic. Over the last two years it has been discovered that Vitamin

B6 is really the complete antidote to nerves. Doctors found that children who had tantrums and were out of control became amicable, happy and easy to manage after they were given a few capsules of Vitamin B6 every day. They then gave it to people in mental homes with very successful results.

But it was Dr. Ellis in Texas who found quite by chance that Vitamin B6 would slim as well. He was treating patients who complained of tingling and numbness in fingers and toes, as well as leg cramp. He gave them fifty milligrams of Vitamin B6 daily.

To his astonishment he found that not only their symptoms disappeared but they also began to lose weight, especially round their waist line, in some cases up to 3″ without changing one element of food in their diets.

It was stated in a medical seminar in Cambridge recently, 'that any woman on the birth pill needs more than "normal" amounts of Vitamin B6 every day' – one of those quite idiotic statements, as I have yet to find any young woman taking Vitamin B6 because they were on the birth pill!

But I am convinced that Vitamin B6 is essential for us all, whatever our age, because it affects our good temper, our sense of well-being and of course our happiness.

Now Vitamin B6, we learn, slims, especially if we combine it with our three other miraculous substances, Lecithin, Cider Vinegar and Kelp.

As I have already said, you can take all these together in one capsule but I do suggest that, to get yourself first down or under the weight you wish to be, you take extra quantities of these four and then go on with the capsules only.

It is so easy and so completely revolutionary that I am very excited at this whole new idea of slimming, which does not make one feel miserable, hungry or depressed.

There is one other thing I would like to suggest as well, which I think one should take at the same time, and that is one Propolis capsule a day.

Propolis, as you know, is the wonderful miracle substance with which the bees seal their hives and which has been proved by a large number of clinical tests in Vienna to be successful when given to people with duodenal ulcers, colitis, and gastric complaints of any sort.

I have found myself that it does prevent any form of indigestion or stomach upsets. Often, when one goes on a new regime, one's inside rebels a little and one might suffer a little discomfort.

I therefore suggest that, besides the four wonderful friends, you take as a chaperon one Propolis capsule a day. The first thing you will notice immediately is that your skin will become clear and more beautiful than you have ever seen it. That is what happened to mine and I have found that whatever I eat there are no upsets, no discomfort, no wind.

So take the four fabulous new friends, all together, and you will be astonished not only with your new, slim, elegant body but also your new, exciting and vivacious personality.

'I shall do exactly what you have told me to do!' Serena exclaimed.

'Good,' I replied, 'I hope everyone does the same, but if you are really over-weight I have a diet which will prove wonderful and bring one's weight down right away, but it must be done carefully.'

'Tell me about it,' Serena said.

'I will explain in another chapter,' I replied, 'because at the moment we must talk about children.'

'Children?' Serena questioned.

'Yes,' I replied, 'because people so often forget that children need attention just as much, if not more, than adults, and as they grow they are often desperately short of Lecithin.

'Incidentally, I've found a Honey which I recommend particularly for people who should feed their nerves. It contains Honey, Sesamine Seeds, and Soya Flour. It really is a complete food, and I'm going to recommend it to all the young men who are working too hard, either at exams or in their businesses, and also to the old people who need some sort of food every four hours.'

'I've heard that Sesamine Seeds are very good,' Serena said.

'They are a most wonderful sustainer of energy,' I replied. 'In the East, when people have to make a long caravan journey across the desert, or go a long period without food, they always put a handful of Sesamine Seeds into their pocket. They know without being told that these seeds contain energy. We know that they are full of vitamins, especially Vitamin B1.'

'I thought Sesamine Seeds were good for sex,' Serena remarked.

'Yes,' I replied, 'they are also tremendously important for all people suffering from sexual difficulties, especially men. Like pumpkin seeds and sunflower seeds, they contain some magic ingredient which does affect a man sexually, and also prolongs his sexual ability into a ripe old age. In many countries of Europe the knowledge of this has been passed down from father to son for centuries, but, of course, we sophisticated idiots are only just beginning to learn about the simple things which primitive people knew instinctively.'

'Honey with Sesamine Seeds sounds delicious,' Serena said, 'I'm marking that down on my list.'

'I forgot to say that it is Mexican Honey—wild Mexican Honey,' I added, 'which, as you know, is collected from the great tracts of unsprayed, unspoilt forest. After the Honey is collected, the swarm just flies away to start making their Honey elsewhere.

'Mexican Honey, I find, is something that men like very much because it isn't over-sweet, and certainly this particular Honey food, which is made by Eustace Miles, is a great favourite with people who haven't got a particularly sweet tooth. Anyway, it's wonderful for nerves, and that is why I suggest that it is taken with Lecithin by those people who feel that life is getting on top of them.'

'And it is very much better for them,' Serena added, 'than tranquillizers.'

She knew this would annoy me, and before I could say any more she said quickly:

'All right, I'm only teasing, but I do know that some people feel they can't face life without something to blunt the edge, so to speak.'

'That is only because their nerves are exposed to all the terrors of modern living,' I snapped, 'and a great deal of it is also psychological. We have got to get it into people's heads that it is no use getting wrinkles all over their face, and grey hair, by worrying about the nuclear and chemical war which may come and again may not.'

'But people do worry about things of that sort,' Serena said. 'A woman said to me last week, "I'm not going to bring any more children into the world so that they can be blown up before they have even begun to enjoy themselves!" '

'That's a pathetically defeatist attitude,' I said. 'Even if we do have to die, we shall yet have had the tremendous and exciting experience of living. I am convinced that this dimension in which we find ourselves now is only a kind of classroom, and the lessons we learn here will always be the same.

'There will always be wars, there will always be interracial problems, there will always be diseases, and, of course, nervous strain. But what we learn from all these things personally is what we are going to carry with us into our next existence, wherever it may be.'

'In other words we have got to live to learn,' Serena said.

'I'm sure of that,' I answered, 'and that is why the parable of the talents is so applicable today. We've got to use our talents, and develop them, enlarge them, and make them bigger and better.

'It's no use hiding them in a handkerchief, or burying them in the ground as the man did in the Bible, or destroying them by taking tranquillizers and sleeping tablets.

'Anything that damages or destroys the brain is the greatest sin of all, because it is through our brain that we learn and that our personality grows.'

'I'm sure you're right about that,' Serena agreed, 'and yet so many people seem to just drift through life not really living, just existing from day to day.'

'Either that, or worrying about a mythical future that

may never happen to them,' I said. 'My father was killed in the First World War, my two brothers died at Dunkirk. None of us can be certain about the future, but it is our job to do our very best to live fully, and we can't do the best for ourselves without trying to do the best for other people.'

'We must use our influence to help and guide,' Serena said quietly.

'Of course,' I answered. 'And everything we say and do, and what we are, affects others. If we show them the wrong image, if we destroy our health, our looks, and our brain, then we are not only harming one particular little person – ourselves – but hundreds, perhaps thousands, of other people, who are affected by us just because we come in contact with them, just because we fail them when they most need our help.'

'That is a very frightening philosophy,' Serena complained.

'But it can also be a very invigorating one,' I replied. 'There is so much for us to do, so much good we can do. But first of all every one of us has to build a foundation of our own health, so that from that foundation we can radiate help and comfort and sustenance to others.'

'I feel you ought to start a crusade,' Serena said with a smile.

'I am fighting one already,' I answered. 'Good health for everyone is the most important fight I have ever undertaken. I've got to make people see that only by being strong and healthy can they combat all the dangers, live through all the problems and difficulties, and conquer all the evils which beset us at this present time.'

'And these are many,' Serena murmured solemnly.

'There is no weapon more powerful than man's imagination and man's faith in himself,' I went on, 'and in something greater than himself. But a miserable, diseased, unhealthy body makes it hard for anyone to believe in all that is beautiful, all that is noble, and all that is fine.'

'That is what we want for our children!' Serena cried.

'This is a crusade,' I continued, 'a crusade against disease and all the evils that attend it. I am convinced that poverty and degradation, war, cruelty, and violence all emanate from unhealthy minds dwelling in unhealthy bodies. It is in good health that we are near to the Divine in whose image we have been made.'

CHAPTER SEVEN

HONEY FOR HAPPINESS

'Which Honey should I use?' Serena asked.

I laughed.

'I think that's the first question everyone asks me after I've been speaking about Honey,' I said. 'Frankly all Honeys are good and any Honey is better than no Honey. As you get more discriminating you'll find that Honey has different flavours, different smells, and different effects, so that it's like choosing a bottle of wine, only it's so very much better for you.'

'But there are so many Honeys on the market,' Serena said. 'When I go into a Health Store I often wonder how people can even begin to make up their minds.'

'That is half the trouble,' I answered. 'People want to learn a little bit about what they are going to buy before they actually get to the shop and feel compelled to make a choice. First of all, let's remember what a wonderful product Honey is. Do you know that a bee makes 2,000 trips to flowers to produce even a thimbleful of Honey, and when you think of the amazing amount of Honey that is produced all over the world, one really feels quite sorry for the bee.'

'I think Honey is getting more and more popular,' Serena observed.

'It must be,' I agreed. 'Every year Australia, for instance, produces between 30 and 50 million pounds of Honey, and about half of this is exported.'

'Besides being eaten, is it used for other purposes?' Serena inquired.

'Oh, it's used in thousands of things,' I said. 'In chewing-gum, in the centre of golf balls, as a preservative of eggs in cold storage, and it can even be used as a powerful anti-freeze mixture in car radiators, because Honey can't freeze and therefore it is a natural aid to our best and most expensive car.'

'Well, let us get back to my first question,' Serena suggested, 'and tell me which Honey I must buy.'

'Well, then I shall start with Honey which is produced in Great Britain,' I answered, 'because I feel that one should always support the home market if it is possible.'

'But Great Britain is full of pesticides,' Serena objected.

'The bees still soldier on,' I answered. 'Do you know that 37,000 loads of nectar have to be carried by bees to produce one pound of Honey? This means travelling from 50,000 to 500,000 miles.'

'Good Heavens!' Serena exclaimed, 'I feel quite sorry for them.'

'It would take a single bee,' I went on, 'about 35 to 40 years to make one pound of Honey! That is why it makes me so angry when people complain that Honey is expensive. There is nothing else which is produced with so much energy, intelligence, and love.'

'It is amazing,' Serena agreed.

'All Honeys help health, but I myself feel that primary or virgin Honey is best, in other words Wild Honey, of which I have already told you. But it is important to go to a reputable firm which really makes an effort not to boil the Honey.'

'Why on earth should they do that?' Serena asked.

'You see, imported from abroad, Honey arrives in large drums of 6 cwt. each with only a small hole in the top. These invariably are full of pieces of wax, as well as perhaps a bit of a bee, a leaf, and other oddments that get into it, especially from primitive countries.'

'It sounds dangerous to health,' Serena suggested.

'Well, actually it's nothing of the sort,' I replied, 'because you know that Honey is sterilizing to any foreign bodies, and is antiseptic as well as being a preservative. So it's perfectly safe, but obviously it doesn't look very pretty. What is more, the Honey in the drum is usually set hard, so it has to be melted to enable it to be pumped out through a strainer.'

'So they have to heat it,' Serena said quickly.

'Of course,' I answered, 'but as long as they get it up to not over 140°F, it does little or no harm to the vitamin value of the Honey. It's a pity it has to be done at all, of course, but I can't see the public being very pleased to see all sorts of foreign bodies in the nice clean jars they buy in the Health Stores. So the Honey is heated for a short period only.'

'But, of course,' Serena said with a smile, 'it's much better to eat Comb Honey.'

'Naturally,' I answered, 'Most of the honey sold in Britain used to be *set* honey, which is made from clear honey by a most mysterious crystallizing process. Recently, more people have been buying *clear* honey, perhaps because it is easier to use in cooking.

'Both are of course extracted from *comb* honey – always an expensive buy, because the small combs offered for sale call for a very high level of bee-keeping skill to achieve their perfect shape.

'With comb honey, you are really getting a whole food, with a guarantee that it has not been tampered with in any way. Most honey varieties are available in set or clear.

'Now, what can we choose from?

'*ALLINSON* offer Mexican honey, one of the deeper flavoured varieties, and with the attraction that it comes from areas where chemical fertilizers are still little used.

'*APPLEFORD* are one of the companies who offer 7lb sizes of honeys, which you can either transfer into smaller pots, or use as they are.

'The big sizes saves you a little on the price, and gives you every encouragement to use honey every day in the kitchen.

'Their choice includes Delicia Honey and Sesame Spread – a delicious spread for bread or topping for yoghurt.

'*FLORAPOLL* are my own favourite choices – Honey Magic, which is a blend of honeys, Hungarian Acacia Clear,

New Zealand Orange Blossom Clear, Guatemalan Clear, Jamaican Logwood Set and Australian Light Amber Set.

'Acacia is noted for its light, beautiful colour and delicate flavour. As I have already told you the colour of a honey is often a guide to the flavour.

'HAPPY FARM produce Rumanian Acacia, Australian, Mexican, New Zealand Clover and Spanish Orange Blossom and Clear.

'They also have Spanish Sunflower, Tasmanian, Pure Blended, Argentine, Canadian Clover, French Heather, Greek Hymettus, Guatemalan Set and Jamaican.

'New Zealand and Canadian Clover Honeys are amongst the most popular of all flower varieties. They set very hard, a texture some people obviously love. The flavour is very delicate and delicious.

'HEATH AND HEATHER have a Honey Special Blend, Greek Hymettus, Rumanian Lime Blossom, Spanish Orange Blossom, New Zealand Clover, Golden Mexican, Canadian Floral, Guatemalan Everyday and Rumanian Acacia.

'Greek Hymettus honey is probably the most luxurious and exotic to most people. After all, it was the food of the Gods!

'It comes from the wild thyme which fills the warm Greek air with an irresistible fragrance.

'Hymettus Honey is always very expensive, but that is because so many people want it, and the Greeks cannot produce vast quantities.

'RATCLIFFE, Britain's largest specialist honey packers, have a list of varieties which is just too long to repeat. But besides almost every honey you can think of, they have some original and very exciting varieties – Tanzanian Wild Bee honey, for instance; Columbian Coffee Flowers, and delightful 'Mini Combs' – whole tiny honeycombs.

'They also offer honey in pottery containers, making an attractive gift. RATCLIFFES make Raw Comb Cappings, which I have already told you about. Some of my friends find it marvellous for Hay Fever.

'ROWSE offer Acacia, Australian, Canadian, Hymettus,

Israeli Orange Blossom, Guatemalan, Lime Blossom, Mexican, New Zealand and Spanish Orange Blossom.

'They also have Tasmanian Leatherwood, New Zealand Blossom, which is one of my favourites, Israeli Flower, Argentine, Canadian Flower, and Sunflower.

'Chunk Honey – which are pieces of honey comb inside a jar of liquid honey, come from New Zealand or California.

'Australia is the world's third largest honey producer, after Argentina and Mexico. Their gum tree varieties, like Leatherwood and Amber, have a fascinating deep flavour.

'Incidentally, the Australian Honey Board, Australia House, Aldwych, London, WC2, will provide anyone with information about honey and recipes.

'WHITEGATES offer Mexican Yucatan, Austrian Clover, Rumanian Acacia, Canadian, Australian Amber, Californian Orange Blossom, Guatemala Wild Forest Flower, and Bulgarian – all in 1 lb and 7 lb sizes.

'This is undoubtedly the cheapest way to cook with honey.

'Besides their lovely honey marmalades, HOLGATES make the more scrumptious Honey Nougat bars, containing fruit and nuts; ALLINSON have new Honey biscuits, made with stoneground flour; SHAWS make the irresistible Honey crunch biscuits; and PREWETTS make Honeybran – a honey date and bran breakfast cereal; which is really good, and also a Honey and Sesame fruit candy bar. There is also Honey Muesli, in 13 oz. and 3 lb sizes.'

CHAPTER EIGHT

HONEY FOR SPECIFIC COMPLAINTS

DIET FOR GOOD HEALTH

I always recommend a certain diet for good health. This really applies to every ailment, and should be used by everybody of every age.

Eat lots of HONEY as it is marvellous for your health and looks. It is not fattening and a tablespoonful taken at night in hot water will make you sleep. You must also eat plenty of protein – meat, fish, eggs, and never touch white sugar or white bread. I also think cows' milk is bad for grown-ups. No coffee, no smoking, no drugs of any sort or aspirin, no milk, no citrus fruit, and NO fruit at all if you have rheumatism or arthritis.

HONEY FOR RHEUMATISM

Anyone suffering from any form of rheumatism should follow the diet above. Add Calcium Pantothenate as I have already described.

Be very careful not to take fruit of any sort at any time, and, of course, alcohol is forbidden, except in very small quantities on special occasions. I am suggesting two lots of treatment, one is much more expensive than the other:

1. *Rheum-Elixir No. 5 of Bio-Strath*
This is really a fantastic cure for all sorts of Rheumatic complaints. It contains Honey and special herbs consisting of: Poplar, Willow, Viburnum, Birch, Spiraea, Rhododen-

dron, Birthwort, Calendula, Periwinkle, Heartsease, Daisy, Nettle, Dandelion, Bryony, Couch Grass, Barberry, Rue and Elder.

Gev-E-Tabs or Cantavite Tablets, 2 a day

Calcium Pantothenate, 4 tablets of 500mg each

Vitamin E – 6 a day (this is essential for rheumatic conditions as it improves the whole circulation of the body.)

Healthcrafts Super Bone Meal – 6 a day.

Celaton Vitamin C – one teaspoonful is over 1 gram. Take one in water night and morning.

Celaton CH3 Tri-Plus – 2 a day.

Ginseng – 400 to 1000 mg. a day.

2. Where it is impossible for anyone to afford the expense of the treatment I have outlined above, I suggest they take a teaspoonful of HONEY in Cider Vinegar with every meal.

Calcium Pantothenate – At least 400 to 500mg a day – after the pain has gone drop to 50mg a day.

Super Brewer's Yeast Tablets – 3 after each meal.

Super Bone Meal – 6 a day.

Devil-brew Tea which removes inflammation from the joints.

HONEY FOR MIGRAINE

No milk, no bread, no starchy foods of any sort.

Chew Honey Comb Cappings as often as possible, 1 Propolis Capsule every day and take HONEY several times a day.

Gev-E-Tabs or Cantavite Tablets – 2 a day

Vitamin A Compleat – 3 a day

Super Bone Meal – 4 a day

Vitamin E Compleat – 600mg a day (This can be 3 or 6 capsules)

Quintessen.

For Hay Fever, take the same diet plus COMFREY TABLETS + NEW ERA'S TISSUE SALTS FOR 'HAY FEVER'.

Having taken Honey and vitamins during the day, last thing at night make a tea of Lime Blossom or Camomile. These two are sedatives on their own.

Add two large teaspoonfuls of Honey to the warm tea and drink when you are in bed.

1 dessertspoonful of Vita-Buerlecithin and I also advise taking 3 Ventrux-Acido for digestion as very often non-sleeping is the result not of insomnia, but of indigestion.

HONEY FOR CONSTIPATION, DIVERTICULITIS, COLITIS AND INDIGESTION

To keep in good health take the following:

2 Tablespoons of Allinson's Bran at breakfast with 'LIVE' Yoghurt and add 1 teaspoonful of liquid Honey.

Night and morning two to three Ventrux-Acido with a teaspoonful of honey in Cider Vinegar.

This will make all the difference to your health and happiness.

HONEY FOR NERVES

Before breakfast take a dessertspoonful of Buerlecithin. Have a good breakfast of eggs and bacon and a large teaspoonful of HONEY. Drink Ginseng Tea, I always drink Ilhwa Korean Ginseng Tea.

Gev-E-Tabs or Cantavite – 2

Celaton CH3 Tri-Plus – 2

Panax Ginseng – 2 400 to 1,000 mg.

Lanes Vitamin E – 2 (200mg) or Healthcraft's 600 mg.

Lunch: Protein – meat or fish or eggs, cheese, fresh green vegetables.

Tea: Dessertspoonful of Honey, Luaka Tea.

Supper: Same as lunch.

Last thing at night take a dessertspoonful of Honey in Lime Tea and you will have deep, happy sleep.

Note: Lime Tea can be bought in bags, by Heath and Heather or Pages. Both at Health Stores.

HONEY FOR ANAEMIA

Floradix and a spoonful of Honey twice a day.

Add Vitamin B_{12} or Intrinsic Factor to your other vitamins.

HONEY FOR HAIR

This is a formula given by Mr. C. E. Tomby of White Gates, who is a great authority on Honey and has a magnificent head of hair:

'The Hair Shampoo for use on brunettes, consists of one third liquid Honey and two thirds pure Olive Oil. The mixture should be stood in hot water just before use in order to facilitate mixing. Shake the bottle well and apply the mixture to the hair and massage by means of a hair-dryer or by getting the head near to a fire. The heat will help the Honey and oil to penetrate the hair and scalp. After twenty minutes or so, wash the hair with a good shampoo. Dry in the normal way.

'Hair will retain its natural colour and lustre for years if treated once a month in this way.'

CHAPTER NINE

'THE WONDER DIET'

'You promised you would tell me about the diet for people who are over-weight,' Serena said, 'and my uncle is over 18 stone at the moment and something has to be done about him.'

'Most men today, because of the lives they lead which we have already discussed, tend to put on fat and are over-weight by the time they are forty.

'One of the most dangerous things is stop—go slimming. A friend of mine who lived on the whole a pretty healthy life, but who drank and ate slightly to excess, used to allow himself to get two or three stone overweight. He then went to a Health Farm to lose a stone in a fortnight and return home to start again.

'The other day at the age of fifty-five he picked up something rather heavy in his garden and fell dead. It was not the fact that he was overweight which killed him, but the fact that he had been doing the dangerous stop—go slimming for quite a considerable time.

'The body's amazing mechanism can adjust itself to a man being fat just as it can adjust itself to a man being rather slim. What it cannot cope with is a man being a kind of see-saw, and it is this which causes heart failure far more often than being too fat.

'One of the best ways for a man to live a normal life and still enjoy the art of eating and a reasonable amount of drinking, is the low carbohydrate diet which has been known for some years, but which has never been as popular as other diets, because it is mainly successful with men.

'Women can lose weight on it, but not so successfully as men do.

'The low carbohydrate diet has been known by many names: "Calories don't Count", was perhaps the most famous, "The Drinking Man's Diet" and now "The Air Force Diet".

'The U.S. Air Force Academy Diet says—"This is a diet designed for those people who have difficulty in losing weight on the usual low-calorie diet. It works by restricting carbohydrate intake, thereby causing the body to burn fat for energy instead."

'It is really very simple, but I want to make quite sure that a man, before he undertakes it, realizes there are certain snags.

'First, no diet should be continued for too long, and I am told that if you go without carbohydrates for too long, it can affect your hearing. As men on the whole go deaf quicker than women, this is important to remember.

'Secondly, the low carbohydrate diet which is very restrictive on vegetables and fruit is constipating. And nothing can be worse for the health of the brain than constipation.

'I therefore advise any man who follows this diet to lose a small amount of weight, say half a stone at a time, give it a rest and then go back to it again.

'In the interval a man should eat reasonably, but not restrict the carbohydrates especially where vegetables are concerned to such an extent that he becomes permanently constipated or finds there are other side effects.

'I still think the best way for a man to lose weight is by exercise. Therefore if he will exercise and follow this diet, he will find an immediate and quick result.'

THE WONDER DIET

This is very simple, it can be summed up in one short sentence. You may only eat 60 grams of carbohydrates a day but – and this is very important – you *must* eat 60 grams.

It is no use thinking you will be clever and cut out carbohydrates altogether, that is dangerous.

Add up what you have ordered and do not exceed the permitted 60 grams, but do not go below 50.

It is estimated that an ordinary diet contains 400 grams of carbohydrates a day. For instance a slice of bread contains 12 grams. One teaspoonful of white sugar is 12, one lump 7.

Sugars are of course the important things to cut anyway. I have already shown how bad white sugar is for you, but unfortunately brown is even higher in carbohydrates than white sugar.

However you will be cheered up to know that a teaspoonful of honey is only 4 grams, so you can have your four teaspoonfuls of honey a day and only use up sixteen of your precious grams.

This diet was called The Drinking Man's Diet because most drinks except beer contain no carbohydrates. But that doesn't mean you can start swilling down the whisky! As I have already told you that is bad for your health and your sex life.

I have made a list of the things you are most likely to want to eat and drink every day, so that it is easy to choose them. Should you however want a more comprehensive list than I can give you in this small book, I would like to recommend *Be Slim and Healthy* by Linda Clark.

Linda is a brilliant American dietician who has studied the whole subject of weight, and her book is well worth reading for any man who wants to have the right type of figure.

One last word. I believe in all sincerity that as one gets older a little extra fat is a protection. I also think that fat people are warmer, more loving, less nervous and neurotic than thin ones. Certainly in a woman a round unlined face is more becoming than a thin wrinkled one.

What you have to discover, if you want to be happy, is the weight at which you are at your best.

You well know what that is because you then wake up in the morning feeling full of energy, you can work full out during the day and enjoy yourself in the evening. This is good health – it is as simple as that.

So don't worry what your tailor, your wife or children say, if you feel a hundred per cent leave yourself alone.

It is only if you get breathless walking up the stairs, if you get a pain under your heart after a large lunch, if you find it is impossible to keep up with your family when you are out for a walk, that you should think about doing something for yourself. That is where the Wonder Diet comes in.

One last point, before starting your diet you should check your general physical condition with your doctor and tell him of your intention to diet.

The Wonder Diet

A		Carbohydrate (grams)
ALMONDS	Shelled, 1 cup	28
APPLE	Medium size	18
APPLE JUICE	1 cup	34
APRICOTS	Fresh	4
	Dried, 1 cup	100
ASPARAGUS	Cut spears, 1 cup	6
AVOCADOS	Half	6

B		
BACON	Two slices	1
BANANAS	Raw	23
BRAZIL NUTS	1 cup	15
BEANS	Broad, 1 cup	29
	Green, 1 cup	6
BEEF	3 oz	0
BEEF STEW	1 cup	15
BEETS	1 cup	16
BISCUITS	Sweet, 1	18

		Carbohydrate
		(grams)
BLACKBERRIES	Raw, 1 cup	19
BLUEBERRIES	Raw, 1 cup	21
BREAD	White, 1 slice	12
	Raisin, 1 slice	12
	Wholemeal, slice	11
BREADCRUMBS	1 cup	65
BROCCOLI SPEARS	1 cup	8
BRUSSEL SPROUTS	1 cup	12
BUTTER	1 pat	Trace

C

CABBAGE	Raw, 1 cup	5
CAKES	Plain, 1 slice	23
	Chocolate, 1 slice	70
	Fruit, 1 slice	17
CANDY	Caramels, 1 oz.	22
	Chocolate, 1 oz.	16
	Fudge, 1 oz.	23
	Boiled sweets, 1 oz.	28
CANTALOUPE	Half	9
CARROTS	Raw, 1	5
CASHEW NUTS	1 cup	35
CAULIFLOWER	Cooked, 1 cup	4
CELERY	One stalk	1
CHEESE	Cheddar, 1 oz.	Trace
	Cottage, 1 oz.	1
	Cream, 1 oz.	1
	And most other cheese	1
CHERRIES	1 cup	15
CHICKEN	Any part	0
CHOCOLATE	1 oz.	16
COCOA	Using milk, 1 cup	26
COLA DRINKS	1 cup	28
COCONUT	1 cup	13
COFFEE	1 cup (no cream)	0

		Carbohydrate
		(grams)
CORNFLAKES	1 oz.	24
CRACKER BISCUITS	1	5
CREAM	Medium, 1 tbs.	1
	Heavy, 1 tbs.	Trace
CUCUMBER	6 slices	1

D

DATES	1 cup	134
DOUGHNUTS	1	17
DUCK	Half pound	0

E

EGGS	Raw, 1	Trace
	Boiled, 2	1
	Scrambled, 1	1

F

FATS	Lard, 1 cup	0
	Veg. Fat, 1 cup	0
FIGS	Raw, 3 figs	22
	Dried, 1 fig	15
FRANKFURTER	1	1
FRUIT COCKTAIL	Canned, 1 cup	50

G

GOOSE	Half pound	0
GOOSEBERRIES	½ cup	9
GRAPEFRUIT	½	14
GRAPEFRUIT JUICE	Fresh, 1 cup	23
GRAPES	1 cup	26
GRAPE JUICE	1 cup	42
GREENS	Cooked, 1 cup	8

		Carbohydrate (grams)
H		
HADDOCK	Fried, 3 oz.	6
HALIBUT	1 serving	0
HAM	3 oz.	1
HEART	Beef, 3 oz.	1
HONEYDEW MELON	¼	8
I		
ICE-CREAM	Plain, ¾ cup	15
J		
JAMS	1 tbs.	14
JELLIES	1 tbs.	13
K		
KIDNEYS	3 oz.	1
L		
LAMB	Any part	0
LEMONS	1	6
LEMON JUICE	Fresh, 1 cup	20
LEMONADE CONCENTRATE	Added water, 1 cup	28
LETTUCE	1 head	6
LIME JUICE	Fresh, 1 cup	22
LIMEADE CONCENTRATE	Added water, 1 cup	27
LIVER	Beef, fried, 2 oz.	6
LOBSTER	Boiled, 1 serving	Trace
LUNCHEON MEAT	2 oz.	1

M		Carbohydrate (grams)
MACARONI	1 cup	32
MACAROONS	1	10
MACKEREL	3 oz.	0
MARGARINE (Vegetable)	1 tbs.	Trace
MAYONNAISE	With Veg. oil, 1 tbs.	Trace
MILK	1 cup	12
	Skimmed, 1 cup	13
MILK BEVERAGES	Cocoa, 1 cup	26
	Malted-milk, 1 cup	32
	Chocolate, 1 cup	27
MILK DESSERTS	Custard, 1 cup	28
	Corn starch, 1 cup	39
MOLASSES (Cane)	1 tbs.	13
MUFFINS	1	19
MUSHROOMS	1 cup	9

N		
NOODLES	1 cup	37

O		
OILS (Vegetable)	1 tbs.	0
OLIVES	12 large	1
ONIONS	1	11
ORANGES	1	16
ORANGE JUICE	Fresh, 1 cup	26
OYSTERS	1 cup	8

P		
PANCAKES	1	8
PARSLEY	1 tbs.	Trace
PARSNIPS	1 cup	12
PEACHES	1	10

PEANUTS	1 tbs.	2
PEARS	1	25
PEAS	1 cup	52
PEPPERS	Raw, 1 pod	3
PICKLES	1	3
PIECRUST	1 crust	72
PINEAPPLE	1 cup	19
PINEAPPLE JUICE	1 cup	32
PHEASANT	Half pound	0
PLUMS	1	7
POPCORN	1 cup	11
PORK	3 oz.	1
PORRIDGE	1 cup	12
POTATOES	1 medium	21
POTATO CRISPS	10 crisps	10
PRUNES	4	19
PRUNE JUICE	1 cup	35
PUMPKIN	1 cup	18

R

RADISHES	4 small	2
RAISINS	1 cup	124
RASPBERRIES	1 cup	17
RHUBARB	1 cup	98
RICE	Puffed, 1 cup	12
	Flakes, 1 cup	26
ROLLS	1	20
RYE WAFERS	1	5

S

SALMON	Pink, canned, 3 oz.	0
SARDINES	3 oz.	1
SAUSAGE	Pork, 4 oz.	0
SHORTBREAD	1	5

		Carbohydrate (grams)
SHRIMP	Canned, 3 oz.	0
SOLE	Grilled, 3 oz.	0
SOUPS (Canned)	Broth and Consommé, 1 cup	0
	Veg., 1 cup	14
	Tomato, 1 cup	18
	Pea, 1 cup	25
	Chicken, 1 cup	10
	Beef, 1 cup	11
SPAGHETTI	1 cup	32
SPINACH	Cooked, 1 cup	6
SPROUTS	Raw, 1 cup	4
SORBET	1 cup	58
STEAK	3 oz.	0
STRAWBERRIES	Raw, 1 cup	13
SUET	1 tbs.	0
SWEETBREADS	1 serving	0
SUGAR	Gran., 1 tbs.	12
	Icing, 1 tbs.	8
	Brown, 1 tbs.	13
SYRUP	1 tbs.	15

T

TANGERINES	1	10
TANGERINE JUICE	1 cup	25
TAPIOCA	1 tbs.	8
TOMATOES	1	6
TOMATO JUICE	1 cup	10
TOMATO KETCHUP	1 tbs.	4
TONGUE	3 oz.	Trace
TRIPE	Beef, 3 oz.	0
TROUT	1 serving	0
TUNA	3 oz.	0
TURKEY	Half pound	0
TEA	1 cup (no cream)	0

V		Carbohydrate (grams)
VEAL	3 oz.	0
VEGETABLE OIL	1 cup	0
VENISON	½ lb	0
VINEGAR	1 tbs.	1

W		
WATER	1 cup	0
WATERMELON	1 wedge	29
WHEAT (Puff)	1 oz.	22
WHEAT GERM	1 cup	34
WHITE SAUCE	1 cup	23
WHITE FISH	1 serving	0

Y		
YEAST	1 oz.	3
YOGHURT	Plain, 1 cup	13

	Alcoholic beverages	Carbohydrate (grams)
ALE, MILD	12 oz.	12
APRICOT BRANDY	1 oz.	6
BEER (Lager)	12 oz.	18
BENEDICTINE	1 oz.	7
BRANDY	1 oz.	0
CHAMPAGNE (Dry)	4 oz.	2
CIDER (Hard)	6 oz.	2
CIDER (Sweet)	1 cup	34
CRÈME DE MENTHE	1 oz.	6
CURAÇAO	1 oz.	6
DAIQUIRI	3 oz.	5
EGGNOG	4 oz.	18

		Carbohydrate (grams)
GIN	1 oz.	0
GIN AND TONIC	10 oz.	9
GINGER ALE	1 cup	21
MARTINI	3 oz.	Trace
MINT JULEP	10 oz.	3
OLD-FASHIONED	4 oz.	4
PORT	2 oz.	7
PLANTER'S PUNCH	10 oz.	8
RUM	1 oz.	0
SHERRY (Dry)	2 oz.	1
SHERRY (Medium)	2 oz.	2
SHERRY (Sweet)	2 oz.	6
TOM COLLINS	10 oz.	9
VERMOUTH (French)	3 oz.	4
VERMOUTH (Italian)	3 oz.	14
VODKA	1 oz.	0
WINE (Dry, White)	4 oz.	0
WINE (Red)	4 oz.	0
WINE (Rose)	4 oz.	1
WINE (Sweet, White)	4 oz.	5
WHISKY	1 oz.	0

For further information, see *The Drinking Man's Diet*, price 34p from Cameron & Company, c/o Allied Graphic Arts Inc. Ltd., 18 Ramillies Place, London W1V 2BA, or see 'Carbohydrate Computer' in *Be Slim and Healthy* by Linda Clark, published by Keats Publishing Inc., New Canaan, Connecticut, U.S.A.

CHAPTER TEN

THE MAGIC OF HONEY

As you know, I have no financial interest in anything I recommend as Health Foods because I believe as President of the National Association for Health I must be completely impartial. But when I was approached to choose six different honeys to be blended together and called HONEY MAGIC, I agreed. This then is my choice and I know it will help people to better health:

Israeli Orange Blossom: 'Honey is gathered from the trees which produce Jaffa oranges and has the reputation of being a nervine – extract from the flowers is used as a carminative in stomach disorders.'

New Zealand Clover: 'Contains fruit sugar in ample quantities and is a speedy source of energy. The natives (Maori) use the honey for chest complaints.'

Hungarian Acacia: 'The Acacia tree blossom provides a honey containing a broad spectrum of trace elements. Much used by athletes as a speedy source of energy.'

Australian Light Amber:	'Gathered from the blossom of the Gum Tree and Mimosa flower. This honey is of value to the food industry as the fine flower does not vary. Used in pharmacy as the basis of cough syrups for its beneficial demulcent properties.'
Guatemalan Clear Honey:	'Gathered from mixed flora and trace elements are well represented including vitamins.'
Jamaican Logwood:	'Renowned for its astringent properties. Therefore, much used as a haemastat. Trace elements found include larger amounts than normal of the B complex vitamins.'

EXTRA HEALTH PRODUCTS WITH HONEY

Bio Ginseng Cream, by Dany Bernard

This is such a perfect cream that it absorbs immediately on the face and it removes wrinkles and of course unsightly scars from the face as it also contains Vitamin E.

Honey Crunch Biscuits, by Shaw

These are my favourite biscuits and they are absolutely delicious. They are made of oats, nuts, molasses, and Yucatan Honey. I've seen in Mexico the lovely wild flowers and trees from which the bees obtain this very subtle Honey.

Obtainable from: Health Stores.

Honey Fudge, by Holgates

This is really delicious and the best Honey fudge I have ever tried.

Obtainable from: Health Stores

Honey Gar, by Martlett

A delicious health drink made with pure honey, blended with Martlett Cider Vinegar.

Honey Ice-cream, by Barbara Cartland

This is my own recipe and we always have it at home. If it doesn't freeze hard and is rather like a cold soufflé, you have put in too much cream.

½ cup fresh or frozen fruit puree (raspberries are best)
¼ cup Honey
1 cup thick cream or yoghurt
Pinch of vegetable sea salt
2 fresh egg whites
1 tablespoon lemon juice

Mix cream (or yoghurt) with fresh or frozen fruit puree. Add fresh lemon juice, Honey, and a pinch of vegetable sea salt: mix thoroughly. Place mixture in freezing tray and freeze until quite firm. Then remove to a bowl and stir until smooth. Beat egg whites until quite stiff and fold them into mixture. Return to freezing tray.

Honey Cup Bev, by Symingtons

A natural Carob substitute for chocolate but without the latter's caffeine content.

Honey Muesli, by Prewetts

Made with organically grown cracked-wheat kernels, oat-flakes, seedless raisins, Honey, skimmed milk powder, chopped hazelnuts, and dried apples. I like this best when it has been soaked overnight and added to a banana or grated apple. Add cream or Fordham Yoghurt.

Obtainable from: Health Stores.

Honey Snaps, by Holgates

When we were children the one thing we loved was Honey Snaps or Brandy Snaps. These by Holgates are adored by all ages and when they come to the Nursery children will find them irresistible.

Honey & Sesame Nu Bar, by Prewetts
One of the famous range of Prewetts Fruit Bars, but sesame is of course rich in natural oil.

Lemon & Honey Drink, by Lanes
A delicious lemon drink with the added flavour of honey which children will love.

Molasses and Honey Drops, and Pineapple and Honey Drops, by Brighton of Hove
Start sucking and you go on and on until the packet is finished. All children like them and they really are made of pure ingredients.
Obtainable from: Health Stores.

Pluss 3, by Applefords
Wonderful for rheumatism, in fact it is very helpful and very cheap.
Obtainable from: Health Stores.

Pure Honey Orange Marmalade, by Holgates
When people come to stay they go into ecstasies over my marmalade. I personally have never eaten anything nicer at breakfast.
Obtainable from: Health Stores.

Young Victoria's Old Fashioned Honey Combed Crunch
Delicious crunchy bars made by Power Health Foods; both children and grown-ups love them.

Welsh Honey Nougat Cymreig, by Holgates
A Welsh delicacy made from pure Honey, nuts, and fruit. It is simply scrumptious and the best nougat I've ever eaten
Obtainable from: Health Stores.

Wheat Germ with Sugar 'n Honey, by Kretschmer Wheat Germ Products

Everyone loves this, it is a sheer delight at any meal. It is an excellent source of Vitamins B and E, and a balanced combination of protein, vitamins, minerals, and nutrients. Perfect for slimming.

Obtainable from: Health Stores.

MEDICINE

Apiregis Gelee Royale, by Ortis

This is excellent for one's health and nice to take in the small glass provided with the bottle.

Obtainable from: Health Stores.

Herb & Honey Cough Mix, by Weleda

This is a natural soother and is quite pleasant to take.

Honey with Fennel Cough Mix, by Salus Haus

This again is very soothing and very effective.

Lavinia Special Foot Cream, by The Natural Health Centre

Contains Bio-Strath and pure Honey. I've given this cream to dozens of friends and they have all been delighted with it. It is excellent for tired, aching feet, chilblains, and sore heels.

Obtainable from: Health Stores or The Natural Health Centre, 147a Ashby High Street, Scunthorpe, Lincs.

COSMETICS

Cucumber Astringent, by Charles Perry

The mild acid reaction of Honey on the skin makes it a natural ingredient of Cucumber Astringent. This is a gentle lotion of freshly extracted cucumber juice, witch hazel, and Honey, with the addition of only just enough vegetable alcohol to dissolve various essential oils. Unlike most astringents, it has not an immediate drying effect, but used after cleansing over a period, it ensures a lovely skin tone and texture.

Obtainable from: Health Stores.

Honey & Iris Toner, Honey & Orange Astringent and Honey & Orange Cleanser, by Weleda
I use all these myself and think they are very good.

Honey Mask, by Scentaflora
This is an easy to apply quick mask to make you look wonderful the same evening. Leave on for a quarter of an hour and you will look a new person.

Honey & Rosemary Foam Bath, by Scentaflora
This neutralizes the hardness of water which dries our skin. It relaxes and is delightfully romantic.

Honey Pollen Cream by Ronald Hagman
A delightful smooth cream which leaves the skin fine and clear yet glowing. Many stage stars swear by it.

Obtainable from: Health Stores and Hagman Laboratories, Beaconsfield Mews, New Southgate, N. 11.

Reform Ginseng and Royal Gelee, by Power Health Foods Ltd.
These have a special quality combined with a magical substance which I find fantastic.

Satilene, by Scentaflora
A satin-smooth cream containing pollen. It makes your skin feel like satin and is suitable for dry and sensitive skins.

Special Antiseptic Cosmetic Lotion, by Charles Perry
Honey, as we've read, was used for the treatment of wounds and skin troubles. It is therefore in this Special Antiseptic Lotion. Intended originally as a cleanser for greasy disordered skins, it has proved effective for many uses. It eases minor burns, sunburn, and insect bites, it is a splendid mouthwash and gargle, and a little rubbed into the

scalp before shampooing will effectively remove dandruff scales.

Obtainable from: Health Stores.

Vitamin Hair Tonic, by Charles Perry

This contains Honey for its nourishing effect on the scalp and hair, and plant extracts such as Nettle, Salvia, and Bayberry Bark, Rosemary and Bay. It is an excellent tonic for stimulating growth and improving the colour, and my sons always use it.

Obtainable from: Health Stores.

Yin Yang Skin Conditioner

This is a scientifically made Skin Conditioner which I find is not only wonderful for the skin but also removes brown age spots from the hands. All the Ying Yan products have special properties which are very rare.

Linomel, by Rayner and Pennycock

This is prepared from whole linseed shredded and blended with pure honey. It is a source of extra energy and increases physical vigour and efficiency. Excellent for children.

Obtainable from Health Stores.

NOTE. If any of these products are not in your Health Store, please ask them to apply to Dietmart Ltd., Fife Road, Kingston, Surrey.

CHAPTER ELEVEN

INDEX OF PRODUCTS MENTIONED
AND ADDRESSES

Page No.

A

ALLINSONS —

Mexican Honey 106

Honey Biscuits 108

Bran 111

Health Stores

APIREGIS ROYAL JELLY – Ortis 129

Health Stores

APPLEFORDS Delicia Honey 106

APPLEFORDS Sesame Spread 106

Health Stores

AUSTRALIAN HONEY BOARD 108

B

BE LOVELY CREAMS 88

Anna Chisholm, 112 Whitehall Court, S.W.1

BIO-STRATH — New Era

Health Stores

Elixir 56 & 57

Rheum-Elixir No. 5 109

BIO-GINSENG CREAM — Dany Bernard 126

Health Stores or

Power Health Foods, 4 Kirkland Street,

Pocklington, York

Page No.

BONE MEAL TABLETS – Healthcrafts   45, 82 & 110
  Health Stores
BRAN   17, 18 & 22
  Health Stores
BREWER'S YEAST SUPER – Healthcrafts   110
  Health Stores

C

CANTAVITE TABLETS   110 & 111
  Cantassium Company, 229 Putney Bridge Road,
  S.W.15
CALCIUM PANTOTHENATE ACID   45, 47, 48, 49, 53, 59,
    109 & 110
CALCIUM PANTOTHENATE INJECTIONS –   53
  Cantassium Co., 229 Putney Bridge Road, S.W.15
CELATON
  Health Stores or
  Biocosmetics Limited, 128 High Street,
  Edgware, Middlesex.
    Celaton CH3   35
    Celaton CH3 Tri-Plus (BRAIN PILL)   30, 31, 32 & 110
    Celaton Day Moisture Cream   88
    Celaton Night Star Special   87
    Celaton Night Star Cream   88
    Celaton Vitamin C   110
CIDER VINEGAR   95, 97, 110 & 111
  Health Stores
COMFREY TABLETS   110
  Rayner & Pennycook, Covett Avenue,
  Shepperton, Middlesex.
CULPEPER
  Health Stores or
  Culpeper Limited, 21 Bruton Street, W.1
    Aperient Tea   62
CYCLAX – Face Powder   86
  Cyclax Ltd., 65 South Molton Street, W.1

F

FLORADIX – Salus Haus   59, 61 & 112
Health Stores

FLORAPOLL HONEYS   106 & 126
Health Stores

FLORAPOLL   39
Health Stores or
Health & Diet Food Co., Freeland House,
Cranleigh, Surrey

FORMULA 3+6 TABLETS (FOUR SLIM FRIENDS)   95
Health Stores or
Health & Diet Food Co., Freeland House,
Cranleigh, Surrey

G

GEV-E-TABS – Healthcrafts   32, 34, 45, 57, 110 & 111
Health Stores

GINSENG   30, 32, 33, 58 & 110
Health Stores

GINSENG TEA – Ilhwa   111
Health Stores
Ilhwa Korean Ginseng Tea, United Family
Enterprises Ltd., Rowlane Farmhouse,
Dunsden, Reading, Berkshire

H

HARMOGEN (H.R.T.)   51
Doctor's Prescription only

HAY FEVER TISSUE SALTS – New Era   111
Health Stores

HAPPY FARM HONEYS   107
Health Stores

HEATH AND HEATHER HONEYS   107
Health Stores

HEALTH AND HAPPINESS CLUB   89
Brook House, 25 High Street, Alton, Hampshire

HERB AND HONEY MIXTURE – Weleda   129
  Health Stores

HOLGATES
  Health Stores
    Honey Fudge   126
    Pure Honey Orange Marmalade   108 & 128
    Honey Snaps   127
    Welsh Honey Nougat Cymreig   108 & 128
    Nectarene Skin Food   84

HONEYBRAN – Prewetts   108
  Health Stores

HONEY CUP BEV – Symingtons   127
  Health Stores

HONEY ICE CREAM RECIPE   127

HONEGAR – Martlett   127
  Health Stores

HONEY COMB CAPPINGS – Rowse   28, 70 & 110
  Health Stores

HONEY CRUNCH BISCUITS – Shaws   108 & 126
  Health Stores

HONEY MASK FM29 – Maria Hornes   85 & 86
  Maria Hornes, 16 Davis Street, W.1

HONEY MASK – Scentaflora   130
  Health Stores or
  Sabenex Ltd., 622 Finchley Road, N.W.11

HONEY & ROSEMARY FOAM BATH – Scentaflora   130
  Health Stores or
  Sabenex Ltd., 622 Finchley Road, N.W.11

HONEY MUESLI – Prewetts   127
  Health Stores

HONEY WITH FENNEL COUGH MIX – Salus Haus   129
  Health Stores

HONEY POLLEN CREAM – Ronald Hagman   84 & 130
  Health Stores or
  Hagman Laboratories, Friern Barnet,
  London, N.11

HONEY & IRIS TONER; HONEY & ORANGE
ASTRINGENT HONEY & ORANGE CLEANSER –
Weleda   130
HORMONE REPLACEMENT TREATMENT   27 & 51
HONEY SNAPS – Holgate   127
    Health Stores

I

INTRINSIC FACTOR – Celaton   31 & 112
    Health Stores or
    Celaton Laboratories, 128 High Street,
    Edgware, Middlesex

K

KELP – Heath & Heather   95 & 97
    Health Stores
KEITAFO BANLON PILLS   30, 31, 32 & 35
    Health Stores or
    Celaton Laboratories, 128 High Street,
    Edgware, Middlesex
KRETSCHMERS WHEAT GERM   129
        With Sugar'n Honey
    Health Stores

L

LAVINIA SPECIAL FOOT CREAM   129
    Health Stores or
    The Natural Health Centre, 147a Ashby
    High Street, Scunthorpe, Lincolnshire
LANES VITAMIN E   111
    Health Stores
LECITHIN   95, 96, 97 & 99
    Health Stores
LECITHIN GRANULES – Lanes   95
    Health Stores

LEMON & HONEY DRINK – Lanes   128
    Health Stores
LINOMEL – Rayner and Pennycock   131
    Health Stores
LUAKA TEA   111
    Health Stores or
    Luaka Tea Company, Station Approach,
    Wokingham, Berkshire

M

MELBROSIA EXECUTIVE   39
    Health Stores
MELBROSIA FOR MEN   38
    Health Stores
MELBROSIA PLD   77 & 78
    Health Stores
MOLASSES AND HONEY DROPS – Brighton of Hove   128
    Health Stores

N

NECTARENE SKIN FOOD – Holgate   84
    Health Stores or
    Holgates Honey Farm, Cadwgan Place,
    Aberayron, Cardiganshire
NEW ERA TISSUE SALTS FOR HAYFEVER   110
    Health Stores or
    New Era Laboratories, 39 Wales Farm Road,
    London W3 6XH

P

PANAX GINSENG   111
    Health Stores or
    English Grains Ltd., Overseal, Burton-on-Trent

PERRY – Charles
  Health Stores or
  155 Pitshanger Lane, Ealing, W.5
    Cucumber Astringent   129
    Special Antiseptic Cosmetic Lotion   130
    Vitamin Hair Tonic   131
PLUSS 3 – Applefords   128
  Health Stores
POLLITABS – Health & Diet Food Co.   37
  Health Stores or
  Health & Diet Food Co., Freeland House,
  Cranleigh, Surrey
PREMARIN (H.R.T.)   51
  Doctor's Prescription only
PREWETTS – Assoc. Health Foods Ltd.
  Health Stores
    Honey Bran   108
    Honey Muesli   108 & 127
    Sesame & Honey Nu-Bar   108 & 128
PROPOLIS – Health & Diet Food Co.   70–3, 98, 99 & 110
  Health Stores or
  Health & Diet Food Limited, Freeland House,
  Cranleigh, Surrey
PURE HONEY CREAM – Mrs. Hilda Conway,   69
  20 Broadwater Down, Tunbridge Wells, Kent
PROGYNOVA (H.R.T.)   51
  Doctor's Prescription only

Q

QUINTESSEN – Healthcrafts   54–8 & 110
  Health Stores

R

RATCLIFFE HONEYS   107
  Health Stores
ROWSE HONEYS   107
  Health Stores

ROWSE HONEY COMB CAPPINGS   107
  Health Stores
REFORM GINSENG – Power Health Foods   164
  Health Stores or
  Power Health Foods Ltd., 4 Kirkland Street,
  Pocklington, Yorkshire

S
SHAWS HONEY CRUNCH BISCUITS   108
  Health Stores
SATILENE – Scentaflora Ltd.   130
  Health Stores or
  Sabenex Ltd., 622 Finchley Road, N.W.11

T
"3+6" – Health & Diet Food Co.   95
  Health Stores or
  Health & Diet Food Co., Freeland House,
  Cranleigh, Surrey

V
VITA-BUERLECITHIN   96 & 111
  Health Stores or
  Celaton Laboratories, 128 High Street,
  Edgware, Middlesex
VENTRUX-ACIDO   111
  Health Stores or
  Health & Diet Food Co., Freeland House,
  Cranleigh, Surrey
VITAMINS – Healthcrafts
  Health Stores
    Vitamin A Super   32, 34, 52 & 70
    Vitamin B-Compleat   82
    Vitamin B2   52
    Vitamin B6   94, 95 & 98
    Vitamin B12   26, 32 & 111

VITAMINS – Healthcrafts (*cont.*)

    Vitamin E   32, 34, 50, 51, 52, 53, 78, 87 & 110

    Vitamin E–Compleat   110

    Vitamin A–Compleat   32, 35 & 110

    VM's   43

VITAMIN FF CREAM – Cantassium   88

  Health Stores or

  Cantassium Company, 229 Putney Bridge Road,

  S.W.15

VITAMIN FF 100 TABLETS – Cantassium   88

  Health Stores or

  Cantassium Company, 229 Putney Bridge Road,

  S.W.15

W

WHEAT GERM OIL – Healthcrafts   35

  Health Stores

WHITEGATE HONEYS   108

  Health Stores

Y

Yin Yang Skin Conditioner   131

  Health Stores or

  Yin Yang Natural Products Ltd.,

  45 Chalton Street, N.W.1

THE FASCINATING FORTIES BY BARBARA CARTLAND

'Forty is the youth of old age and the old age of youth' and it is a time when you can combine vitality and beauty with experience and wisdom.

For everyone who believes that to be attractive is the prerogative of youth, here is a book that highlights the triumph of the 'fascinating Forties'. Only with maturity comes charm, poise, glamour, and the spiritual and sexual fulfilment that contribute to the creation of a beautiful woman . . .'

Barbara Cartland, playright, lecturer, novelist, T.V. personality, and President of the National Association for Health, is a dynamic example of the fact that age sets no limits on beauty, vivacity and style. In THE FASCINATING FORTIES she offers encouragement and down-to-earth practical advice for all those approaching what can be the most exciting period of their lives . . .

0 552 09169 3   30p

FOOD FOR LOVE BY BARBARA CARTLAND

Throughout history man has searched for a food to increase and sustain his virility. For the sake of love he has consumed such delicacies as sea urchins, sparrows' eggs, river snails, lizards and hedgehogs. But now the amorous gourmet need no longer suffer these gastronomic tortures . . .

Barbara Cartland has compiled an appetizing selection of recipes – each one specially chosen for its qualities as an aphrodisiac. Such delicious recipes as – Sole in Champagne; Chicken with Orange Surprise; Cucumber and Cheese Mousse; Iced Avocado and Crab Soup and Almond Peaches . . .

All these and more will bring excitement into your cooking – and spice into your life! . . .

0 552 09735 7   40p

THE DIET BOOK FOR DIET HATERS BY DEREK MANLEY

The reasons for excess weight . . . the effortless way to lose that weight . . .

How the diet works . . . the value of foods . . .

All the foods and snacks you can eat . . . and the foods you must avoid . . .

A BOOK FOR THE DIETER – WHO ENJOYS GOOD FOOD.

0 552 10339 X   50p

EAT, DRINK AND BE SLIM BY ANNE SKIMMING

If you have ever wondered in despair how you can become slim, and *stay* slim, without having to stick to a dreary diet and give up all the things you like best, this is the book for you.

Anne Skimming outlines a sensible eating plan, based simply on limiting your carbohydrate intake to 50 or 60 grams a day, whilst allowing you to choose from a wide variety of interesting foods. This book provides a useful table of the carbohydrate values in everyday foods, so you can keep a check on what you eat, menus for 21 days, and a wide selection of delicious recipes which will allow you to eat well – even exotically – whilst remaining within the 60 gram limit.

0 552 10212 1   60p

A SELECTION OF DIET, HEALTH AND COOKERY BOOKS PUBLISHED BY CORGI BOOKS

☐	09735 7	**FOOD FOR LOVE**	*Barbara Cartland* 40p
☐	09292 4	**LOVE, LIFE AND SEX**	*Barbara Cartland* 40p
☐	09169 3	**THE FASCINATING FORTIES**	*Barbara Cartland* 30p
☐	76417 5	**MEN ARE WONDERFUL**	*Barbara Cartland* 25p
☐	10066 8	**THE MAGIC OF HONEY COOK BOOK**	*Barbara Cartland* 50p
☐	10339 X	**THE DIET BOOK FOR DIET HATERS**	*Derek Manley* 50p
☐	10212 1	**EAT, DRINK AND BE SLIM**	*Anne Skimming* 60p